D0718971

00401215521

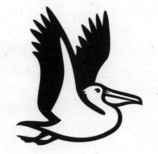

DAVID SPIEGELHALTER AND
ANTHONY MASTERS

Covid by Numbers
Making Sense of the Pandemic with Data

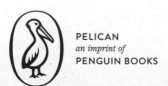

PELICAN
an imprint of
PENGUIN BOOKS

First published 2021
001

Text copyright © David Spiegelhalter, Anthony
Masters, 2021

The moral right of the authors has been asserted

Set in 10/14.664pt FreightText Pro
Typeset by Jouve (UK), Milton Keynes
Printed and bound in Great Britain by
Clays Ltd, Elcograf S.p.A.

The authorized representative in the EEA is
Penguin Random House Ireland, Morrison
Chambers, 32 Nassau Street, Dublin D02 YH68

A CIP catalogue record for this book is available
from the British Library

ISBN: 978-0-241-54773-1

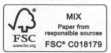

MIX
Paper from
responsible sources
FSC® C018179

Penguin Random House is committed to a
sustainable future for our business, our readers
and our planet. This book is made from Forest
Stewardship Council® certified paper.

www.greenpenguin.co.uk

Contents

Acknowledgements

This book is about statistics, and statistics are often about people. And there are many people who have helped and encouraged us.

Our collaboration grew out of our joint work for the Royal Statistical Society Covid-19 Task Force, and then Robert Yates's request for a statistical column in The *Observer*.

We thank Laura Stickney of Penguin for commissioning the book, helping us forge the outline, and having faith in us to deliver on time. Sam Fulton, Ruth Pietroni, Matt Hutchinson and Julie Woon at Penguin have managed the production and publicity in record time, and Linden Lawson expertly copy-edited our prose. Great credit goes to Jonathan Pegg for looking after us so well.

We want to thank everyone who read chapters, offering thoughts, feedback and improvements, including Arthur Barnett, Sheila Bird, Michael Blastland, Simon Briscoe, Kate Bull, Peter Diggle, Christl Donnelly, Stephen Evans, Kate Fiveash, Scott Heald, Maria Mapletoft, Theresa Marteau, Ruth McCabe, Brian Spiegelhalter, Ruth Studley, Alain Vuylsteke and Stian Westlake. Special thanks go to Kevin McConway, who gave up a huge amount of time to help us. Of course, we take full responsibility for what has finally appeared.

Such a book would be impossible without data. Throughout this pandemic, analysts in organizations have published data and statistics, greatly enhancing public understanding, including Our World in Data, Public Health England, the Office for National Statistics, the army of researchers who have contributed to SAGE reports, the *Financial Times*, *The Economist* and numerous others.

Data visualization is another important pillar of pandemic reporting, and we have taken great inspiration from the work of the BBC and *Financial Times* data-visualization teams. We also want to extend our gratitude as statisticians to everyone who maintains R packages, including Hadley Wickham and the RStudio team, Matthew Kay, Thomas Lin Pedersen and Claus Wilke.

There are many people whose insights with data we have found valuable in formulating this book, including John Burn-Murdoch, Clare Griffiths, Pouria Hadjibagheri, Emma Hodcroft, Oliver Johnson, Meaghan Kall, Christina Pagel, Hannah Ritchie, James Ward, and the whole team at More or Less. The fine team at the Science Media Centre have been central in improving the coverage of the pandemic by bringing together scientists and journalists.

Anthony would like to thank his partner, Samantha Fiveash, for continuing love and support. David has the same deep gratitude to Kate Bull, who has exhibited tolerance beyond the call of duty.

CHAPTER 1

Introduction

Life changed in March 2020, and everyone has their story to tell: the family struggling to home-school their young children, with both parents working from home; the single parent in a tower block without support; the retired middle-class couple missing meals with friends – and their grand-children; the nurse having to work long shifts in full personal protective equipment (PPE); the shopkeeper forced to close down; unemployed young people and teenagers with gap years ruined, stuck at home with their parents; the older person in a care home unable to hug their family; many of us with a nagging sense of unease about how to behave.

Those are the healthy. There is also the young adult fatigued and 'brain-fogged' months after catching Covid-19; the middle-aged man in intensive care without visitors; the relative who dies, amid health-care staff in full PPE, their family denied a fitting funeral.

So many personal stories. But there is another way of understanding what has gone on: by putting all those individual experiences together to form a bigger picture. Counts and measurements are stories writ large, made into statistics and graphs presented to us daily by politicians, scientists and journalists. The data become evidence in arguments in newspaper columns and on social media about lockdowns, risks, vaccines and more.

This book is about all those numbers.

What has happened in the UK?

Never have we as a society been more bombarded by graphs and statistics, and Figure 1–1 summarizes some of what we have been told about the pandemic up to May 2021.

Cases confirmed by a test (A) showed relatively small but rising numbers in March 2020, although limited testing at the time means the number of confirmed cases did not accurately reflect the extent of the spread of the virus. That was swiftly followed by a rapid growth in hospital admissions (B), with deaths (C) exhibiting a similar, but delayed, pattern to admissions. After a peak in early April 2020, steady improvement saw a summer of reduced restrictions. In autumn, improved testing picked up another rise, inexorably followed by more hospitalizations and deaths.

A second lockdown in November was followed by a small dip. The 'tier' system was wrecked (along with family Christmas) by the home-grown Alpha (B.1.1.7, or VOC-20212/01) variant that originated in Kent. After a third lockdown, the measures peaked and started to improve. The successful vaccine roll-out (D) brought a faster decline in hospitalizations and deaths than seen in the first wave. At this point the Delta (B.1.617.2) variant, first identified in India, was yet to have an impact.

Although they would have a different shape, graphs like Figure 1–1 could be drawn for any country with a good surveillance system and the UK has been well served in this respect.

Better tracked with more testing, confirmed Covid cases peaked in the second winter wave

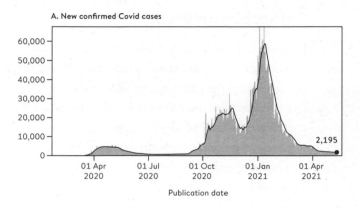

A. New confirmed Covid cases

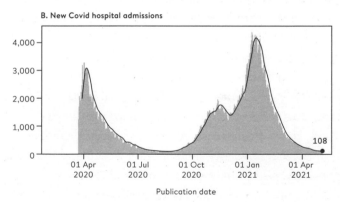

B. New Covid hospital admissions

Figure 1–1

Summary of Covid-19 surveillance measures for the UK reported on each day between February 2020 and 10 May 2021. Seven-day rolling averages are shown – there are lags between publication and occurrence. Deaths are those within 28 days of a positive test.

Source: Public Health England COVID-19 dashboard data download

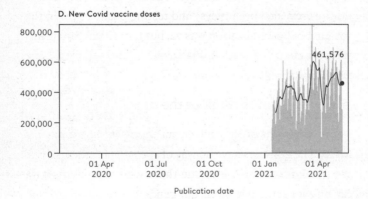

C. New confirmed Covid deaths

1.500

1.000

500

0

01 Apr
2020

01 Jul
2020

01 Oct
2020

01 Jan
2021

01 Apr
2021

10

Publication date

D. New Covid vaccine doses

800,000

600,000

400,000

200,000

0

01 Apr
2020

01 Jul
2020

01 Oct
2020

01 Jan
2021

01 Apr
2021

461,576

Publication date

Remarkably, the US found itself without a functioning national system: volunteers had to start the COVID Tracking Project to collate data from individual states,[2] only ending in March 2021 after better official federal data had come online.

Who has been affected?

A common theme in this book is that detail matters – we need to go beyond averages to personalize the statistics. Another running theme is the importance of age as a vital risk factor: Table 1–1 shows some simple summaries of the ages of those who experienced various events in the second wave starting in September 2020.

Exploring the table reveals estimated typical ages at each level of severity of the disease. The **median** age of infection (as revealed by surveys) and testing positive was in the 30s, that of hospitalization was 72, but for critical care it was younger, at 61. For death it was 83, only slightly above the age for other causes.

Is it enough just to look at the data?

No. In the words of Nate Silver, author of *The Signal and the Noise*, 'The numbers have no way of speaking for themselves. We speak for them. We imbue them with meaning.'[3] Data can answer some questions but generate even more. Young people get infected, but why are so few hospitalized? Why do a comparatively young and narrow band of people end up in critical care? If Covid-19 is so bad, why is the typical age at death about the same as normal?

We will try to find the answers to these and other questions, but comprehension is not always helped by the many

Event experienced in the second wave	Estimated median age of those experiencing event	Estimated age range containing 80% of people experiencing event
Being alive	39	7 to 72
Getting infected with SARS-CoV-2	33	11 to 67
Getting a positive test for Covid-19	37	15 to 69
Being hospitalised with Covid-19	72	34 to 82
Going into critical care with Covid-19	61	43 to 75
Dying with Covid-19 on their death certificate	83	65 to 93
Dying without Covid-19 on their death certificate	82	59 to 92

Table 1–1
Estimated summaries of ages of those experiencing different events in England and Wales in the second wave. If we lined up everyone who had experienced each event in order of their age, the median age would be that of the person halfway along. The 80% range would cover everyone except the bottom 10% and the top 10%. The median age of everyone alive was 39 – this is, quite literally, middle-aged.*

---

* The average age in the population (the **mean**, obtained by adding all the ages and dividing by the number of people) is 41. The most 'popular' age in 2019 (the **mode**, the year group containing the highest number of people) was 53, although all years from 47 to 54 are close contenders.

ways in which data can be presented, for example the alternative displays of Covid-19 deaths shown in Figure 1–2.

Daily media accounts of Covid-19 deaths (A) have an erratic profile driven by reporting delays, which can be smoothed by a seven-day **rolling average*** (B).

We would expect more deaths from a larger country. Rates per 100,000 people (C) give us a similar profile of the European countries in the first wave, with the UK following Italy by around two weeks, then a smaller summer dip in the US and an elongated second wave in Italy.

The final plot shows a **logarithmic scale** (D), in which the gap between 10 and 100 is the same as 100 and 1,000. Such scales have been widely used but not widely understood, yet they can be useful for comparing trends, as '**exponential growth**'† or decline become straight lines. The rates of increase of all three countries were similar in the first wave, while the UK's steep decline from the second wave stands out.

Once again, these statistics can generate their own stories and questions. For example, what is meant by a 'Covid-19 death'? Were these deaths *with* Covid-19 or deaths *from* Covid-19? Was it the vaccine roll-out that explains the difference in outcomes in the UK and Italy?

---

* For each day, this plots the average (mean) of the counts on the day, the three days before it and the three days after it.

† The term 'exponential' simply means that the numbers are increasing or decreasing by a fixed proportion in a fixed period. Exponential growth does not have to be rapid: compound interest of 0.1% per year, as currently available in some savings accounts, still provides exponential (if slow) growth.

There are different ways of showing statistics for reported Covid deaths

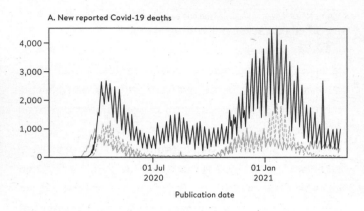

A. New reported Covid-19 deaths

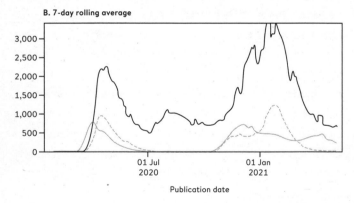

B. 7-day rolling average

Figure 1–2

Alternative ways of visualizing Covid-19 deaths reported by Italy, the UK and the US.[4]

—— Italy   ----- United Kingdom   —— United States

Source: Our World in Data Coronavirus data explorer (Johns Hopkins University CSSE Covid-19 Data)

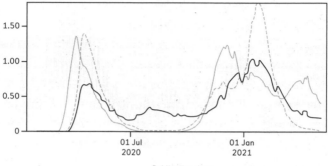

C. 7-day rolling average per 100,000 people

Publication date

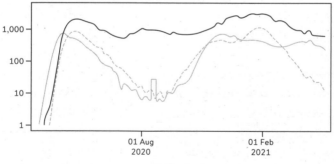

D. 7-day rolling average, on a log scale

Publication date

The structure of this book reflects the kinds of questions asked throughout the pandemic. We start with the virus itself, how it spreads, how infectious it is and the rise of variants, with the focus on statistical summaries and measurements rather than biology. We move on to diagnosis and cases, looking at the quality and use of diagnostic tests, the numbers of confirmed cases and the problem of estimating how many actual infections occur.

Progressing to how the virus affects people, we consider how many get ill and how they recover. This pandemic put enormous strain on the health services and their staff, so we look at what has happened in hospitals and the huge advances in treatments.

We consider death counts, clarifying different definitions, showing how age and sex matter and examining personal risk. We point out the care needed in comparing countries and drawing analogies with past epidemics and other hazards.

One controversial aspect of the pandemic has been the effectiveness of non-vaccine measures such as face masks, lockdowns or contact-tracing. We look at collateral effects, positive and negative, how behaviour has changed and economic consequences. The pandemic has affected our feelings as well as our bodies, so we examine changing beliefs about the risks posed by the virus, the role of misinformation on social media, and the impact on mental health and well-being.

We then come to some good news: the effectiveness and safety of vaccines, and who gets them first. And we look at attempts to produce mathematical models of the epidemic and, with the benefit of hindsight, how projections matched reality.

The future remains uncertain, so we finish by considering some possible paths, without claiming to know which one will come about.

Like viruses, misunderstandings and misinformation can spread through a community, and the pandemic has spawned many false assertions purporting to have a statistical basis. There are good websites that provide detailed arguments against such claims,[5] but we will correct a few, including the notion that most positive tests have been false-positives (Chapter 6), most Covid-19 deaths were 'with' Covid-19 rather 'from' Covid-19 (Chapter 11), Covid-19 is no more lethal than flu (Chapter 12), and excess deaths are caused by the lockdown itself (Chapter 14).

We need to make some apologies in advance. We have had to be concise, and so doubtless your particular interest might not get the attention it deserves. While the whole world has been affected, we mainly focus on the United Kingdom. Each nation in the UK has a different public health system, and there are three different national statistics agencies, which may use different definitions; unfortunately we cannot give all equal attention.

This book is not a critique of policy decisions. We leave it to others to establish what could have been done better, although in the Postscript we draw some statistical lessons from this last year.

While the discussion about the pandemic has been awash

with data, we have written this book because we believe that better attention to statistical issues could have improved understanding. So we make no apology for emphasizing the need for clarity as to what the data refer to, the value of communicating uncertainty and limitations, the need for humility regarding causal claims and the vital importance of rigorous evaluation of interventions.

Finally, a lot more will have happened by the time this book is published and read. But we hope, with the benefit of hindsight, that it can provide a strong statistical perspective on what we have all been through in the first year of the pandemic. While numbers can't answer all our questions, we believe they can raise the quality of the discussion.

The Virus

How did the pandemic develop?

The story of SARS-CoV-2 began in Wuhan, in the Hubei province of China.[1] Within three months of its first identification, civil life across the world changed radically.

What happened up to the first UK lockdown on 23 March 2020?

- **Late December 2019:** there are media reports of 'pneumonia of unknown cause',[2] with a cluster of cases linked to a seafood market in Wuhan.
- **9 January 2020:** the World Health Organization (WHO) reports that Chinese authorities determine it is a novel coronavirus.*
- **11 January:** Scientists publish the genetic sequence of the novel coronavirus.[3]

---

* Viruses have a genome often composed of a strand of ribonucleic acid (RNA) encased in an envelope of proteins, and coronaviruses are distinguished by their crown-like surfaces. They are hardly rare; before 2020 there were six known coronaviruses that could infect humans, four of which cause mild to moderate disease, including common colds. The other two are much more severe: Severe Acute Respiratory Syndrome (SARS) was identified in 2002, and Middle East Respiratory Syndrome (MERS) in 2012.

- **13 January:** The first testing protocol is published.[4] Thailand reports a confirmed case, the first outside China.
- **14 January:** With 41 confirmed cases in China, the WHO says human-to-human transmission is 'certainly possible'.
- **24 January:** France informs the WHO of three cases, the first in Europe.
- **29 January:** Two people in a York hotel report a dry cough and fever after having travelled from Wuhan – the first recorded cases in the UK.[5]
- **30 January:** The WHO declares a public health emergency of international concern. Outside China, it reports 98 cases in 18 countries, but no deaths. China now has over 8,000 lab-confirmed cases and 171 reported fatalities.[6]
- **11 February:** The WHO names the virus SARS-CoV-2, while the disease caused by the virus is Covid-19 (Coronavirus disease 2019).
- **29 February:** Total reported cases reach 23 in the UK.[7]
- **6 March:** Public health agencies report the first UK Covid-19 death.

Figure 2–1
New reported Covid-19 cases and deaths (from any cause following a positive test) in the UK, by publication date. Six government responses are shown by dates with dotted lines.

1   Contain, delay, research and mitigate plan published
2   PM holds first press conference on Covid-19
3   New self-isolation rules for those with symptoms
4   Daily press conferences and social distancing start
5   Schools in England close for most children
6   PM issues stay-at-home order (lockdown begins)

Source: Public Health England Covid-19 dashboard data download

The first reported UK Covid-19 death was on 6 March 2020

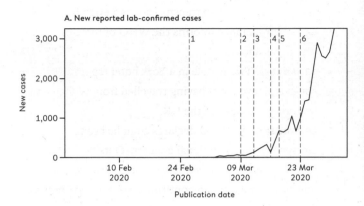

A. New reported lab-confirmed cases

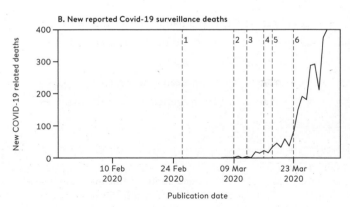

B. New reported Covid-19 surveillance deaths

- **11 March:** The WHO declares a global pandemic.

Our focus now turns to the UK. Figure 2–1 shows that total confirmed cases exceeded 100 on 5 March and 1,000 on 14 March, while deaths reached 100 by 18 March and then 1,000 nine days later.

As cases and deaths rose, government responses evolved.[8] On 26 February the Health Secretary, Matt Hancock, described a plan to 'contain, delay, research, and mitigate'. On 9 March, Prime Minister Boris Johnson held the first Covid-19 press conference, joined by Professor Chris Whitty (Chief Medical Officer) and Professor Sir Patrick Vallance (Chief Scientific Advisor).* Two days later, the Budget pledged supportive measures.[9]

On 12 March, the government announced new self-isolation requirements for people with symptoms. The day after, local elections due in May were postponed: around this time the true urgency appears to have become clear to those in government.[10] By 16 March daily press briefings started, with announcements of 'social distancing' rules. The WHO said there were more confirmed cases outside China than within.[11] Imperial College London published a report estimating, without mitigation measures, around 510,000 deaths in Great Britain and warning that a lack of strict suppression 'would still likely result in hundreds of thousands of deaths and health systems being overwhelmed many times over'.[12]

Two days later, the PM announced that schools in

---

* On 3 March Boris Johnson announced that he had 'shaken hands with everybody' after visiting a ward of Covid-19 patients. Coincidentally, on the same day DS was on BBC's *Newsnight*, and, along with the other guests, did not shake hands with the staff.

England would close for most children. The press briefing on 20 March declared closure of bars, restaurants and other businesses. On 22 March there were new measures for shielding the vulnerable. Finally, on 23 March, there was the Prime Minister's stay-at-home order,[13] calling Covid-19 'the biggest threat this country has faced for decades'.

What became clear in hindsight?

Public health surveillance is incomplete. The first UK death occurred on 30 January 2020 to someone who had never travelled abroad.[14] With mainly hospital-based testing, the number of confirmed cases severely understated the size of the problem; instead of the reported 1,000 cases a day around the time of the lockdown, models later estimated there were around 70,000 or even about 360,000 new infections each day.[*15]

Instead of one outbreak, reverberating outwards like an explosion, we now know there were many occurring simultaneously, with genomic sequencing identifying over 1,000

---

* For 23 March 2020, the London School of Hygiene and Tropical Medicine model estimated about 71,000 new infections (with an interval of 26,000–145,000). The Imperial College London model estimated around 364,000 new infections (338,000–400,000).

[Following pages] Figure 2–2
Statistical estimates of the day of importation of lineages with observerd onwards transmission (imputed) from the lag model. Statistical assignment to each country is a point estimate: there is uncertainty around each of these estimates. Total estimates are rounded.

Source: Establishment and lineage dynamics of the SARS-CoV-2 epidemic in the UK (Science, 2021)

About 6 in 10 imported lineages came from France, Italy and Spain

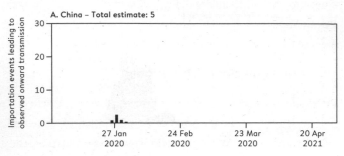

A. China – Total estimate: 5

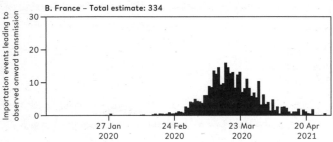

B. France – Total estimate: 334

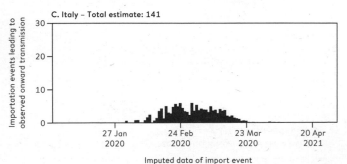

C. Italy – Total estimate: 141

Imputed data of import event

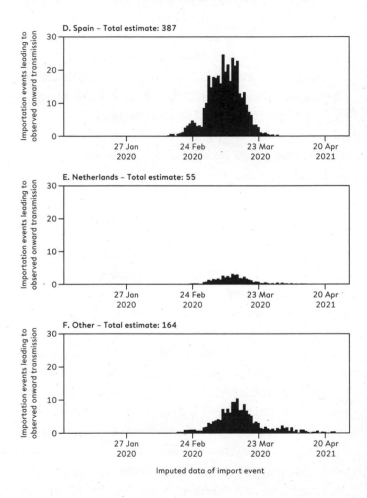

D. Spain – Total estimate: 387

E. Netherlands – Total estimate: 55

F. Other – Total estimate: 164

Imputed data of import event

different seeds of SARS-CoV-2 introduced in early 2020.[16] Figure 2–2 shows there were far more imports of SARS-CoV-2 from France, Italy and Spain than from China, with the peak around mid-March, well after the school half-term but a popular holiday time for adults. This is a statistical assignment, and there is uncertainty: viruses can take indirect flights.

When considering Spanish importations, note that at the Champions League football match at Anfield between Liverpool and Atlético Madrid on 10 March,[17] 49,000 local supporters mixed with 3,000 fans of the opposing team,* while in Madrid schools were shut[18] and supporters could not attend matches.[19]

As the pandemic receded in 2020 some restrictions eased; for example, pubs and restaurants reopened on 4 July. Afterwards, there were greater differences in government responses within the UK. Mandatory masking in shops started on 24 July in England. By September 2020 testing had increased, with rising confirmed Covid-19 cases, particularly in younger people.[20] The virus spread into older age groups, and in response new rules came in force for England: the 'rule of six' (14 September), 10 p.m. closing time for pubs and restaurants (24 September), legal self-isolation orders (28 September), and three-tiered local restrictions (14 October).

It was not enough. A new lockdown in England began on 5 November, ending on 2 December. Rapid rises in cases in south-east England, driven by a new variant, led to a surprise fourth tier (20 December). There was a brief relaxation

---

* To add insult to injury, Liverpool lost 3–2; 4–2 on aggregate.

of rules on Christmas Day, with some divergence between UK nations.[21] The government statement at the time said: 'A smaller Christmas is a safer Christmas, and a shorter Christmas is a safer Christmas.'

Following Christmas a third lockdown began, with vaccinations rolling out. A 'roadmap' for easing restrictions continued.[22]

Different countries around the world followed different paths, and some have suffered more than others. Crucially, outbreaks were scattered across the UK, overwhelming tracing efforts based on limited testing. Arguments will continue about how earlier action could have saved lives, and we return to this issue in Chapter 16.

By June 2021, when we finished editing this book, cases were again rising sharply in the UK, although the link to hospitalization and deaths had been weakened by the vaccine rollout. There was an opportunity to examine what had happened the previous year, and just how dangerous this virus turned out to be.

How infectious is SARS-CoV-2?

A virus can only replicate inside cells of other living organisms; whether it can be considered 'alive' is a philosophical question. At the core of the SARS-CoV-2 virus lies a strand of **RNA** that contains instructions for reproducing the virus. Laboratory studies suggest a full replication cycle of around 10 hours.[*][1] The virus is physically small: one estimate says that all the SARS-CoV-2 virus in the world at one time could fit into a single can of soft drink.[2]

At the start of the pandemic in March 2020, fear of infection from expired droplets on surfaces ('fomite transmission') led to huge emphasis on sanitizing and handwashing, possibly while singing 'Happy Birthday' twice. It is now accepted that the primary route is 'aerosol transmission' from the breath of infected people,[†][3] a classic example being when

---

[*] A single replication cycle can produce 1,000 virus particles, so in the right circumstances the virus effectively doubles every hour, since 2^{10} is about 1,000. So, in principle, it could multiply over a millionfold each day and a trillionfold in two days – this is an extraordinary example of exponential growth.

[†] On 20 March 2020 the WHO claimed that 'Covid was NOT airborne', and that 'Current evidence suggests that the main way the virus spreads is by respiratory droplets among people who are in close contact with each other.' This was only changed more than a year later, on 30 April 2021. The UK government's 'Hands, Face, Space' mantra was eventually changed to 'Hands, Face, Space, Fresh Air' at the end of March 2021.

24 out of 68 passengers were infected during one trip in an unventilated coach.[4] Ventilation and face coverings became far more important.

When is someone infectious?

Figure 3–1 indicates that viral load and infectiousness rise at about the time any symptoms develop, although people can be infectious before developing symptoms – 'pre-symptomatic transmission'. Viral loads tend to be higher in those with more severe symptoms, while people with no symptoms can infect others but are less likely to.[5]

Another important feature is people can continue to 'shed' detectable remnants of RNA – the building blocks of the virus – for days and even weeks after the infectious period.[6] Although not infectious, they could come out positive with a sensitive diagnostic test, prompting unnecessary isolation (see Chapter 5 and Chapter 16).

How infectious is SAR-CoV-2?

We've all had to become familiar with the term 'R', which is the average number of people we would expect someone carrying the virus to infect. First, R_0 (R-zero) is the **basic reproduction number**, which summarizes the infectiousness of the virus in a population in which all are susceptible and no precautions are taken. For the original 'wild-type' SARS-CoV-2, R_0 has been estimated at about 2.9 (2.4–3.4).[7]

Figure 3–2 shows the implications of R_0 equal to 3. With around five days between each stage, this virus can quickly rip through unprotected populations. As the number of infected people multiplies with each stage, the total exponentially

Viral load and infectiousness rise as symptoms develop

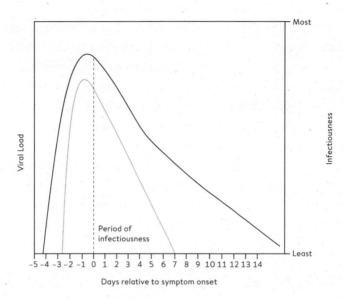

Figure 3–1

A rough impression of the typical period of infectiousness for symptomatic adults, and viral load, adapted from Meyerowitz.[8]

——— Viral load   ——— Infectiousness

Each case spreads to – on average – three people each

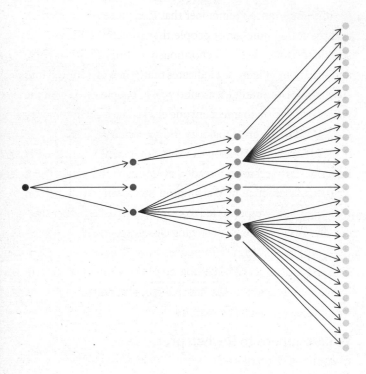

Figure 3–2
An illustration of how a virus with a basic reproduction number of 3 might spread from person to person over three reproductive stages. R_0 is an average, and so the actual number infected will vary.[9]

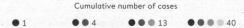

increases, so small changes in R can have a big impact. As we shall see in Chapter 16, modelling suggests that one week's delay in bringing in protective measures might have made huge differences.

It is important to remember that R_0 represents an average, and the actual number of people that someone infects – the secondary cases – will vary enormously according to the people and situation.[10] Figure 3–3 indicates that, when introduced into susceptible communities, around 75% of people who catch the virus do not go on to infect anyone else, while a small minority (10%) lead to the great majority (80%) of new cases.

There are several reasons for this. Some may be particularly infectious, while 'super-spreader' events can also occur. There was a choir practice in Washington State where one person with 'cold-like' symptoms led to 52 infections* of 60 other singers after over two hours of singing closely together.[11]

Prolonged proximity increases risk, although the **absolute risk** can appear low compared to the virus's reputation: infected individuals are estimated to infect around one in six members of the same household.[12]

What happens to R when protective measures are taken?

The basic reproduction number R_0 holds for a 'virgin' population, where everyone is susceptible and nobody takes protective measures. As people develop immunity through past

---

* The Centers for Disease Control and Prevention (CDC) reports there were 30 confirmed and 22 probable infections with symptomatic Covid-19 from a single symptomatic case. Three people were hospitalized, and two died.

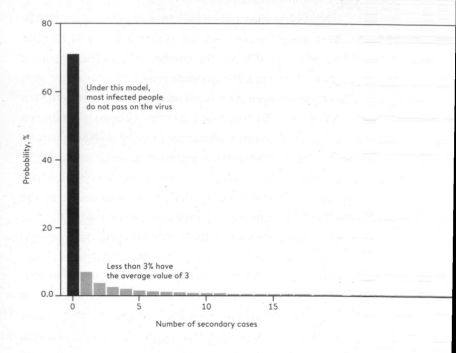

This is a possible distribution of secondary cases of Covid-19

Under this model, most infected people do not pass on the virus

Less than 3% have the average value of 3

Probability, %

Number of secondary cases

Figure 3–3
Estimated distribution of the number of people infected from a single individual in an unprotected community, assuming a mean (R₀) of 3 and a dispersion parameter (k) of 0.1. This distribution has an average of 3, but it is highly unlikely that exactly three people are infected.

Source: Estimating the overdispersion in Covid-19 transmission using outbreak sizes outside China (Wellcome Open Research, 2020)

infection or vaccination and change their behaviour, what matters is the **effective reproduction number**. This number is known as R_t: the average number of secondary cases in the current circumstances.

If R_t is less than 1, then each 'round' of infections will be smaller than the previous one. If that is sustained, the epidemic withers. If R_t is 1, the number of cases stays stable. If R_t is greater than 1, the epidemic grows.

There has been great focus on the current average R_t, but we cannot count transmissions taking place and so cannot directly 'see' R_t. Any estimates are therefore highly uncertain. In the UK there are eight independent teams attempting this challenging task, using broadly similar data sources but different mathematical models; they meet online at the SPI-M-O* committee and agree a consensus range.

Figure 3–4 shows how these consensus intervals changed over the pandemic. This range was confidently less than 1 after the first lockdown,[13] and then the R_t range increased to well above 1 during autumn, before being brought back down below 1 by the November lockdown. With the new variant spreading, the range rose – falling after the third lockdown. By the end of March 2021, the effective range reached its lowest recorded interval of 0.6 to 0.8, and then started to creep up as measures were relaxed.

When does 'herd immunity' occur?

Suppose R_0 is 3 so, on average, an infected person could be expected to meet and infect three people in a society full

---

* Scientific Pandemic Influenza Group on Modelling, Operational sub-group.

The estimated range of the reproduction number in England fluctuates over time

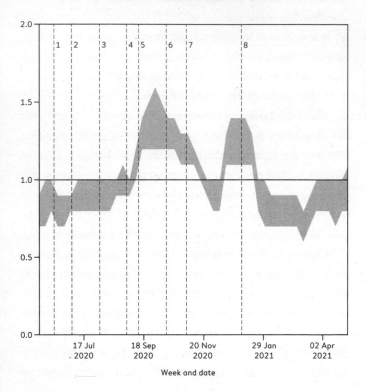

Figure 3–4
Consensus ranges for current reproduction number in England from May 2020 to April 2021.

1 Shops reopen
2 Pubs and restaurants re-open
3 Eat Out to Help Out starts
4 Schools reopen
5 'Rule of six' begins
6 English tiers introduced
7 Second national lockdown starts
8 Third national lockdown starts

Source: The R value and growth rate in England 30 April 2021

of susceptible people. Suppose two in three of people they come across are immune. On average, only one will then be infected, so the effective reproduction number R_t is 1.

This is the classical idea of 'herd immunity', reached when R_t is less than 1. In theory, herd immunity is reached when only $1/R_0$ are susceptible, and so $1 - 1/R_0$ are immune. If R_0 is 3, we therefore need $1 - 1/3$ (67%) to be immune.

Other diseases are rather different.[14] Seasonal flu has an R_0 of around 1.3, and so theoretical herd immunity is achieved if 23% are immune through previous infection or vaccination. Measles is extraordinarily infectious, with an R_0 of up to 18. To protect against measles, around 94% of the population need to be vaccinated. That is why mass vaccination campaigns are so essential.

This equation is a huge simplification of reality! In practice, variation in social activity tends to reduce the necessary proportion of immunity,[15] while limited individual immunity often has the opposite effect.

There have been claims that herd immunity has been, or will soon be, reached, but at the time of writing we are not there yet. A successful vaccine roll-out should – eventually – produce sufficient immunity that, when added to the effect of past infection, should bring the national R_t below one. Even without restrictions, that should prevent any widespread outbreaks, although communities without good protection remain vulnerable.

It is clearly in all our interests that a good degree of immunity is as widespread as possible, whether from infection or vaccination. But then new variants of the virus come along and disturb this process.

What is the risk from new variants?

For every replication of the strand of RNA comprising the core of SAR-CoV-2, there is a tiny probability of a copying or a deletion error. Compared to the original virus, every mistake constitutes a 'variant', and the more the virus is circulating, the more variants will be generated. Small differences are often inconsequential, but sometimes the virus changes in a way that allows it to spread more easily or become more harmful. Another danger is that new variants might also allow reinfection or make protection from vaccines less effective.

Public health agencies investigate variants with troubling properties, and label important ones as Variants of Concern (VOC).[1] In December 2020,[2] the rising Alpha lineage (B.1.1.7) instigated new restrictions across south-east England, introducing a surprise tier, summarily called 'Stay at Home'.[3] That variant had taken hold in the multiple prisons on the Isle of Sheppey and became known as the 'UK variant' in other countries, and the 'Kent variant' in the UK.*[4] By May 2021,[5]

---

* It is unclear what people in Kent called it.

more than 240,000 Alpha (B.1.1.7) cases were confirmed through genomic sequencing.[*]

Why was this variant so concerning? Analysis in March 2021 suggested the Alpha (B.1.1.7) variant was between 43% and 90% more transmissible than other variants,[6] and researchers later estimated it was 61% (42%–82%) more deadly than pre-existing variants.[7] For every three deaths within 28 days of confirmed cases with **wild-type SARS-CoV-2**, there would be about five after Alpha (B.1.1.7) infections.

Using a proxy measure rather than full genome sequencing,[†] the share of confirmed cases with this variant grew fast, from 7% around mid-November 2020 to 94% by the end of January 2021.[8] Figure 4–1 shows its rapid climb to dominance in other countries, for example rising from 4% of Denmark's SARS-CoV-2 cases in early 2021 to 75% seven weeks later.[9]

Many other variants are of interest or concern. Beta (B.1.351) was first identified in South Africa in October 2020,[10] becoming the dominant variant in that country, while Gamma (P.1), found in Japan among travellers from Brazil, led to a rapid growth in Covid-19 hospitalizations in Manaus, with reported reinfections among health-care workers.

---

[*] A genome – an organism's genetic material – is like an instruction manual, written in a special code of four nucleotide base 'letters'. Human DNA is about 3 billion base letters long. In contrast, SARS-CoV-2 has a short RNA strand of around 30,000 letters. Researchers can 'read' these letters in a process called sequencing.

[†] Standard testing involves detecting certain genes, generally the three ORF1ab, N, and S, representing different parts of the coronavirus, and a positive test finds at least one of these genes, excluding the spike protein (S-gene) on its own. The Alpha (B.1.1.7) variant has deletions in the spike protein at positions 69 and 70, which causes standard tests to fail to detect the S-gene, and so spike-gene target failure (SGTF) can be used as a proxy measure for the new variant.

The Alpha variant rose to dominate sequences in several countries

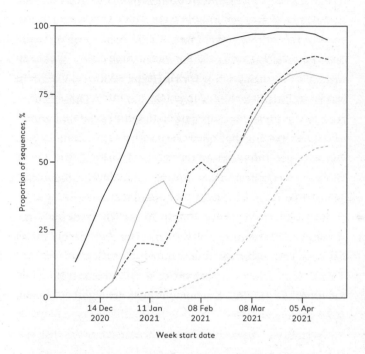

Figure 4–1
For each country, the proportion of sequences which are the Alpha (B.1.1.7) variant. Sequences may not be a representative sample of cases in each country.

——— UK ----- Italy ——— Spain ----- USA

Source: CoVariants (GISAID)

In May 2021, the Delta (B.1.617.2) variant became a Variant of Concern* and started to dominate Alpha (B.1.1.7) in some regions. The **secondary attack rate** (**SAR**) is an impressive term for a simple idea: the proportion of an infected person's contacts who also get infected. Using NHS Test and Trace data for recent non-travel cases, Public Health England estimated the secondary attack rate for the Alpha (B.1.1.7) variant was 8.1% (+/- 0.2%), while for the Delta (B.1617.2) variant it was substantially higher at 13.5% (+/- 1.0%).†[11] These figures are likely to understate the true values due to the limitations of contact-tracing, but again emphasize that a minority of contacts get infected. At the time of writing, the Delta (B.1.617.2) variant appears a formidable development and generates even more uncertainty about the future.

Effective surveillance is important for tracking viral spread and this contest of variants, but fortunately there has been extraordinary international scientific cooperation. Thanks to its laboratory capacity, the UK has contributed to the global SARS-CoV-2 genome repository about a quarter of its sequences.[12]

Variants will inevitably continue to appear. As we shall see in Chapter 22, there are reasonable expectations that vaccines will either cope with variants or be adaptable. This will be important as we learn to live with the virus.

---

* Media reports used the phrase 'double mutant' to describe the B.1.617 lineages. That phrase is meant to refer to two mutations in the spike protein (E484Q and L452R). Since viruses have lots of mutations, the term does not have a specific meaning.

† Here, the **confidence interval** of the Delta (B.1617.2) variant's secondary attack rate was 12.5%–14.6%. It reflects uncertainty in the central estimate.

Diagnosis and Cases

How good are diagnostic tests?

The popular idea of a diagnostic test is straightforward:

1. somebody either has a disease or not
2. they take a test which comes out either positive or negative
3. that test tells us the truth.

The reality is rather more complicated, made worse by ambiguous terms and unintuitive results, and this makes the area a minefield for the unwary (and means this chapter is rather more challenging than most).

First, there are different definitions for a 'true-positive' case. Does it mean they carry the virus, or the virus is capable of replicating, or they are infectious? In general, the first, broadest definition is used.

Second, the tests in regular use vary in what they call a 'positive' result, whether they are laboratory-based reverse transcription-polymerase chain reaction (PCR) tests, or rapid lateral flow devices (LFD).

Third, all these tests can give 'wrong' results: false-negatives (which could lead to false reassurance and possible spread); or false-positives (which could lead to unnecessary concern and isolation).

What is a positive test?

In PCR testing,[1] laboratory technicians add enzymes to a swab sample from a person's nose or throat. Those enzymes convert strands of the viral genetic material to a DNA copy, which is then repeatedly amplified with the aim of detecting specific parts of the SARS-CoV-2 virus, like a game of 'Guess Who?'.

The **cycle threshold** (Ct) is the number of times scientists need to do this molecular photocopying to reach detection, so that *high* Ct values correspond to *weak* concentrations of genetic material, associated with lower viral load and risks of infectiousness.[2] It could also mean a degraded sample, or the person is in the early stages of infection, or non-viable viral fragments after the person stopped being infectious.[3] Unfortunately, there is no standardization across laboratories, which may use different gene targets and cycle threshold limits.[4]

The Office for National Statistics (ONS) Covid-19 Infection Survey categorizes positive tests into 'higher', 'moderate' and 'lower' evidence, using gene detection, cycle thresholds, symptoms and place of work.*[5] Usually most positives are 'higher evidence', but at times of low prevalence the few

---

* *Higher evidence*: two or three genes detected, irrespective of Ct value. *Moderate evidence*: single gene detection if the Ct value was less than 34 or if there was a higher pre-test probability of infection (any symptoms at or around the test, or reporting working in a patient-facing health-care role or resident-facing care-home role). *Lower evidence*: all other positive tests, which were therefore all in asymptomatic individuals not having a patient-facing or resident-facing role with a single gene detected with a Ct value of 34 or higher.

detected infections tended to be weaker, with higher Ct values. By late July 2020, the proportion of 'higher evidence' positives fell from above 80% to less than 30%.[6] Indeed, when there is little virus in circulation, the UK government guidance requires tests that were only positive at the 'limits of detection' to be repeated before confirmation of a case.[7]

Lateral flow device tests put a liquid nasal or saliva sample on an absorbent pad, along which the liquid flows, and can give a result in 30 minutes.[8] There is a strip with antibodies which bind to the proteins of the SARS-CoV-2 virus: if these proteins are present there is a coloured line, although the precise properties will differ between manufacturers. This is how pregnancy tests operate, but instead of expecting a baby you may expect to self-isolate.

How accurate are the tests?

The accuracy of a diagnostic test is characterized by two quantities. The 'true-positive rate' is the proportion of people with the virus who get a positive result, called **sensitivity**. The 'true-negative rate' is the proportion of uninfected people who get a negative test, also known as **specificity**. Discussion is more often in terms of false-positive rates (100% minus specificity) and false-negative rates (100% minus sensitivity).

At the end of June 2020, less than 0.05% of ONS Covid-19 Infection Survey PCR tests were positive.[9] This means that, even were there no circulating virus, the estimated false-positive rate could not be more than 0.05%, and the ONS estimates it to be closer to 0.005%.[10] So out of 20,000 people without the virus, we would only expect one to test positive. For the same procedure, the false-negative rate is likely to lie between 5% and 15%, so between 85% and 95% of infected people will test positive. These figures may not hold under different testing regimes: for example, it may depend on who takes the sample, and whether individuals are being re-tested as a check.

When it comes to rapid lateral flow device tests,[11] a review found that they are most accurate for those with symptoms, but PCR tests are the 'gold standard'. Of people with confirmed Covid-19, the true-positive rate (sensitivity) was 72% for those with symptoms but 58% for those without. For people who were PCR-negative, the true-negative rate of rapid tests among symptomatic people was 99.5%, and for those without symptoms it was 98.9%. Different brands of devices had different accuracy; with the Innova test, post-marketing surveillance in March 2021 suggested that around three to 10 in 10,000 uninfected people get a positive result, meaning a specificity of 99.90%–99.97%.[12]

Rapid lateral flow device tests miss some people with the virus, although hopefully they pick up many infectious cases, while having a low false-positive rate.

How accurate are the conclusions of the test?

Rather than knowing how the tests perform on groups of people with and without the virus, people want to know what the result means for them as individuals. For example, if you test positive, what is the chance you are infected? These are the **predictive values** of a test.

Suppose a lateral flow test has a true-positive rate of 60% and a true-negative rate of 99.9% (a false-positive rate of one in 1,000), and the virus is at the level it was in early March 2021, when around 0.3% of the population had an infection. Figure 5–1 shows what we would expect to happen if we test a million people.

Three thousand people have the infection, and so we get 1,800 true-positive results (60% of 3,000). Of 997,000 uninfected people, 997 (0.1%) get a false-positive result. The proportion of true-positive results of all positives is about 64% (1,800 divided by the sum of 1,800 and 997).*

The false-positive rate is one in 1,000, and yet 36% of positive results are false. This can be confusing, to say the least.[13]

As the virus gets rarer, more positive results will be false – when you think you have found a needle in a haystack, be prepared to be wrong.

What are the roles of tests?

Tests serve multiple purposes. They can be used for population surveillance, to determine the probability of how many people have a condition, as in the ONS Covid-19 Infection Survey. Or they can be used for making decisions about individuals, either for 'red-light' testing, as a dragnet to find as many cases as possible, or 'green-light' testing (or 'testing to enable'), when negative tests allow people to take part in normal activities.

---

* This is an application of **Bayes' Theorem**, which shows that the underlying prevalence of the condition is vital in interpreting the results of the test.

Illustrative frequency tree of diagnostic test results when prevalence is low

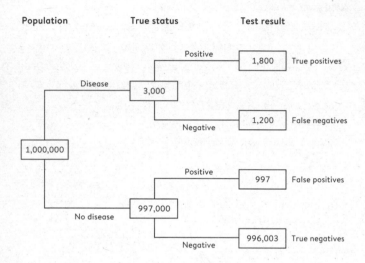

Figure 5–1

'Frequency tree' showing what we could expect if we tested 1,000,000 people in which 0.3% have the virus. The test is assumed to have a sensitivity of 60% (detects 60% of cases of people who have the virus) and a specificity of 99.9% (1 in 1,000 people without the virus will get a false-positive test result).

Requiring someone to isolate with a false- or post-infectious positive test is unnecessary. Allowing an infected person into schools or other places could be dangerous. There is a continuum of risk, through which repeated rapid testing can provide a hazy guiding light. In the next chapter, we see what has happened in practice.

How many cases have been found?

Every day, news reports announce the number of new recorded Covid-19 cases. What can we learn from these figures?

In general, we only hear about cases confirmed by a positive test.* Although there is no requirement to have symptoms, public health agencies might only test people with symptoms, so cases are biased towards more severe disease. It is clear that the case numbers we hear about are an undercount of those who are actually infected (we cover this in Chapter 7).

By 30 April 2021,[1] total reported cases reached 151 million worldwide. Figure 6–1 shows the broad shape in four continents, with European countries reporting about 45 million and North America about 38 million cases, with large winter spikes. Vaccination programmes hastened the decline from these peaks.

In contrast, Asia and South America showed increasing numbers of confirmed cases. Those in Africa remained

---

* The European Centre for Disease Control (ECDC) allows for three levels of confidence about cases: *possible* shows consistent symptoms; *probable* indicates symptoms after a confirmed contact or which meet diagnostic imaging criteria: *confirmed* is a positive laboratory test result.

Europe and North America recorded high numbers of cases over the winter of 2020

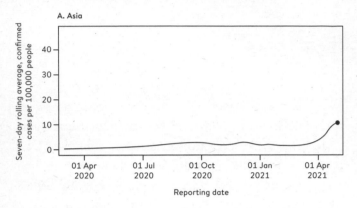

A. Asia

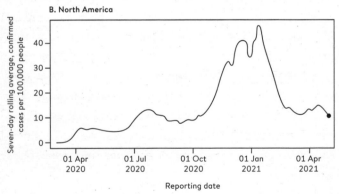

B. North America

Figure 6–1

Seven-day rolling average of confirmed cases per 100,000 people in four continents between 1 March 2020 and 30 April 2021.

Source: Our World in Data Coronavirus Data Explorer

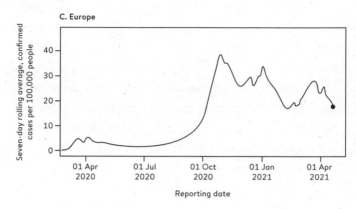

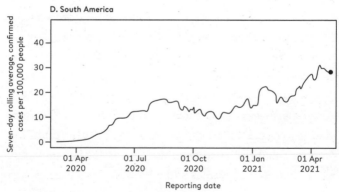

subdued, declining from 2.4 per 100,000 people in January to 0.8 by the end of April.

But great caution is needed when comparing claimed case rates from different countries, which can differ by availability, eligibility and types of test. At one extreme, countries may just stop counting. In June 2020, the late President Magufuli of Tanzania declared the country 'coronavirus-free',[2] and after that Tanzania did not report a single confirmed case.* Edicts may ease the statistical collection process but do not inspire confidence in accuracy – Turkmenistan and North Korea have also not reported any Covid-19 cases.

Figure 6–2 and Table 6–1 summarize both the size of the testing operation and what has been found in the UK.†

Figure 6–2 (A) shows that, after a slow start, the UK PCR testing regime grew steadily throughout 2020, with 90 million conducted in the UK up to mid-May 2021. Lateral flow device tests (B) started in 2021, rising to an average of over a million a day around mid-March after schools reopened. There was a peak of over 2 million on 28 March before meeting people outdoors was permitted. Over 70 million of these rapid tests had been used by early May, including 8.9 million in care homes and 27 million for students and staff in secondary schools.[3] Tests were freely available to the public, although their benefit was unclear (see Chapter 16).

---

* President Magufuli died in March 2021.

† These combine counts from testing in Pillar 1 (those with clinical need and health and social workers), Pillar 2 (general public) and Pillar 4 (research purposes). Pillar 3 are antibody tests.

Covid testing expanded in the UK, with many lab and rapid tests being done each day

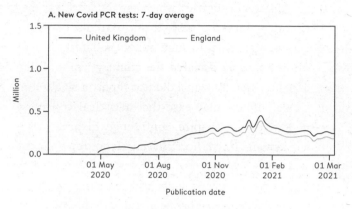

A. New Covid PCR tests: 7-day average

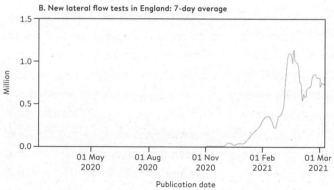

B. New lateral flow tests in England: 7-day average

Figure 6–2

Covid-19 testing metrics in UK and England by publication date (PCR and LFD tests, 7-day averages) and specimen date (positivity)

Source: Public Health England COVID-19 dashboard data download

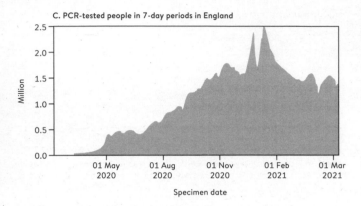

C. PCR-tested people in 7-day periods in England

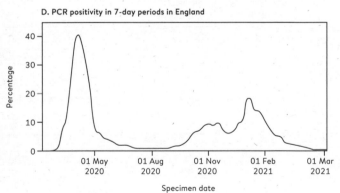

D. PCR positivity in 7-day periods in England

Area		Total confirmed cases	Cases per 100,000 people
UK		4.474 million	6,700
Highest Local Authority	Blackburn with Darwen	19,334	12,920
Lowest Local Authority	Orkney	74	330

Table 6–1
Confirmed cases in the UK up to 26 May 2021. (Case rates are rounded to the nearest 10.)

In the week ending 28 April 2021, secondary-school students registered taking 1.4 million LFD tests at home, of which only around 1,300 came out positive (0.1%). Of about 500 matched to a later PCR test, 40% came back negative. This high false-positive share among those getting a positive LFD test is very similar to the example in Chapter 5, which explains why confirmatory PCR testing is sensible when the virus is rare.

Figure 6–2 (C) shows a peak of 2.5 million people getting a PCR test in England in the first week of January – around one in 20 of the population provided a swab. Figure 6–2 (D) reveals that in England,[4] the **positivity** – the proportion of PCR tests with positive results – peaked at over 40% in the first week of April 2020. At the start of the pandemic, testing was mainly kept for patients with severe symptoms, and such high positivity rates suggest a large pool of undiagnosed cases. As testing capacity rose and stabilized, patterns of positivity mirrored patterns of cases.

Table 6–1 summarizes UK confirmed cases, showing that around one in 16 of the entire population had been confirmed as a case by mid-May 2021. Rates varied across the country: the highest are about double the national average, and Orkney is somewhat of an outlier.

India carried out 2 million tests per day in late May 2021. In a population of 1.4 billion, that means that only one in 700 was tested – around a tenth of the UK rate.[5] In early May, 20% of Indian tests were positive, indicating many unconfirmed cases.

Was there a 'case-demic'?

There are several reasons why confirmed cases would be an *undercount* of the true number of infections. There have also been claims that, because of false-positives, confirmed cases are an *overcount* and the rise in autumn 2020 was just a 'case-demic'.

That theory rested on the observation in Chapter 5 that at times of low prevalence, many positives would be either false or 'lower-confidence' ones. That is why – in those circumstances – the guidance recommends further confirmatory testing for positive PCR tests at the limit of detection.[6] Also, for a period from October 2020, confirmed cases in England included all positive results from lateral flow devices. On 9 April 2021, Public Health England removed positive rapid tests where the confirmatory PCR test returned negative. This change reduced the cumulative total by over 8,000 cases.[7]

But, while there certainly can be many false-positives when the virus is rare, the subsequent rise in hospitalizations and deaths from all causes in the autumn and winter of 2020 exposed the case-demic hypothesis as ill-founded.

How many people have been infected with SARS-CoV-2?

Put simply, we do not know. Many people will have been infected and be unaware or untested, and so the number of 'confirmed cases' is bound to be an underestimate. To seek better answers to key questions such as how many people are infected, or how many got infected today, or how many ever caught the virus, we rely on that old tool – the **sample survey**. In the words of the statistician John Tukey, it is better to get an approximate answer to the right question (by doing a good survey) than get a precise answer to the wrong question (counting confirmed cases).

The basic idea is that we only need a sample to understand the whole population, provided the sample is representative. One key way in which to gather a representative sample is through choosing people at random. In the memorable image of the survey researcher George Gallup, you do not need to eat a whole pot of soup to find if it needs more salt: you only need a spoonful, *provided it has been stirred well*.

The ONS began recruiting participants for a survey in April 2020. Through an extraordinary effort, they published the first results in three weeks.[1] A year later, the survey had involved following up over 450,000 individuals from 230,000 households, with a total of over 4 million PCR tests.[2] It was a massive endeavour.[*3]

The acceptance rate in England for the first two waves was about 44%, and households who agreed to take part would not have been completely representative.[†4] Data from under-represented groups are **weighted** up, but some biases could remain. Other studies include the REACT-1[5] survey[‡] and the ZOE Covid Symptom Study app,[6] which has over 4.5 million contributors. These studies get similar answers to the ONS survey, providing valuable cross-checks.

How many people have it at any one time (the prevalence)?

All the nose or throat swabs in the ONS survey are subject-ed to PCR tests and declared positive or negative. Raw data goes through sophisticated **statistical modelling**, adjusting for imbalances in the participants, and provides an estimate of the proportion of the population that would test positive. This is shown in Figure 7–1 from when the survey results started in May 2020, with **margins of sampling error**. Because the PCR test is imperfect, these figures do not directly represent the proportion of infected people – the true prevalence.

---

* Participants received at least £25 in vouchers for each swab. By the end of January 2021, 116,000 vouchers worth £3.8 million had not been redeemed and had subsequently expired.

† Participants in previous ONS surveys were originally invited. The acceptance rate dropped to 16% when additionally sampling random addresses.

‡ This involves around 150,000 participants each month taking swab tests to determine prevalence at a single point in time, without follow-up.

The trend in positivity differs between the nations

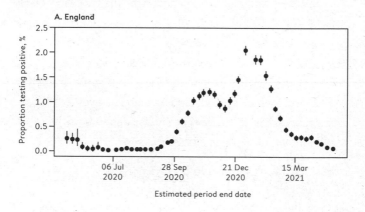

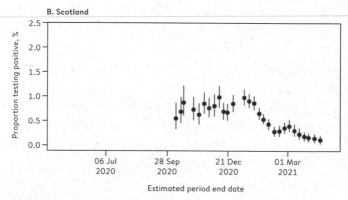

Figure 7–1

Estimated proportions of the community that would test positive
for SARS-CoV-2 in nations of the UK between May 2020 and
April 2021; 95% uncertainty intervals are narrower for England,
as the sample size is greater. These figures do not include those in
institutions such as hospitals, care homes and prisons.

Source: Office for National Statistics – Covid-19 infection survey

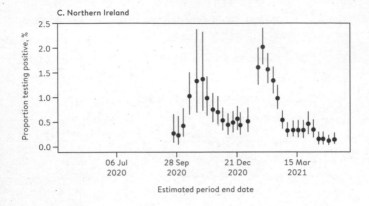

C. Northern Ireland

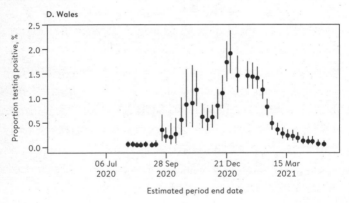

D. Wales

The four nations followed a slightly different pattern, but the peak was around the start of 2021: one in 50 of the community would have tested positive, over a million people in the UK. In contrast, rates were extremely low in summer 2020 and spring 2021. In the six weeks from 31 July to 10 September 2020, out of over 200,000 swab tests only 159 were considered positive (0.08%). We saw in Chapter 5 that, when prevalence is low, these positives tend to have high Ct values and are likely to be less infectious.[7]

These rates are averages: the chance of an individual getting infected will depend on their contacts and precautions. Some occupations increase viral exposure, and the ONS provided estimates of the raw positivity rates of 254 occupational groups over the second wave between September 2020 and January 2021.[8] In this period, an average of 4% of the working population (one in 25) tested positive, but limited numbers in specific groups prevent precise comparisons. It is notable that paramedics and ambulance staff ranked top, with 12% testing positive, despite the availability of protective gear. For outdoor occupations, none of the 93 sampled street cleaners, forestry or farm workers tested positive over this four-month period.* We shall see in Chapter 13 that Covid-19 death rates have varied substantially across occupations.

---

* Out of 213 paramedics and ambulance staff sampled, 25 tested positive over these four months, which gives a 95% uncertainty interval of 8%–17%, well above the average. The uncertainty interval for 0 out of 93 outdoor workers is 0%–5%. In general, error margins for individual occupations are wide, making definitive ranking unreliable. These positivity rates were not adjusted for other risk factors.

How many have been catching it each day (the incidence)?

It is challenging to estimate the incidence rate – the proportion of the community catching the virus each day – but it can provide an idea of how much the number of reported daily cases undercounts those actually infected. With repeated tests on the same individuals, the ONS produce a modelled estimate that rose and fell like the case numbers in Chapter 1. Estimated incidence reached a maximum at Christmas 2020, when around one in 500 people in England were getting infected each day (99,100–115,400 individuals). The minimum came in July 2020, with about one in 30,000 people per day (around 1,700).* Rates were probably higher back in March 2020, but the survey had not started then.

After Christmas 2020, around 50,000 new cases were being reported each day,[9] compared to the ONS estimate that about 100,000 new people a day would have tested positive, although that latter figure does not include hospitals or care homes. That suggests a rule of thumb: less than half of infected people make it into the published case numbers.

How many have antibodies after catching Covid-19?

Antibody tests provide another way of monitoring who has had, possibly unknowingly, an infection.

---

* This figure used an unweighted estimate from the weekly midpoint. Incidence estimates changed to Bayesian modelling later, leading to some incomparability with earlier estimates.

The virus consists of an RNA genome coated in a protein 'bag'. These proteins constitute antigens, which the immune system recognizes as 'foreign'. On first encounter, our immune system takes some time to build up its initial response, mounting its attack by targeting the structural antigens of the viral coating. Those responses include the production of circulating antibodies, which can be measured in blood samples. Like all diagnostic tests, the antibody test is not a perfect measure. The blood sample may be too small, or the response too limited, to provoke a positive test result.

In early December 2020, before vaccines started contributing to the immunity in the population, the ONS estimated that around 13% (10%–16%) of the English population had antibodies, corresponding to about 7 million people having survived a previous infection.[10] These rates dropped steeply with age: the ONS estimated that 25% (18%–36%) of those aged between 16 and 24 had antibodies, compared with only 3% (1.5%–5%) of over 80s, suggesting high levels of undetected infection in younger groups.

Antibody tests do not give a complete picture of our immune capacity. Our 'adaptive' immune system is complex, comprising both B-cells (antibody-producing cells) and T-cells (whose activity does not show up on these tests). Both 'remember' the viral antigen (whether met through previous infection or vaccination), and so get triggered when exposed again.[11] Mounting an effective second response is quicker.

An optimistic lobby asserted that previous infection by other coronaviruses (including common colds) conferred protection against SARS-CoV-2, enabling much less stringent anti-virus measures.[12] The crashing experience of multiple waves of infection countered these claims of high proportions of pre-existing immunity.

Although around one in five of the population* had been infected by May 2021,[13] it became clear that an effective vaccination programme was essential to bring outbreak-limiting immunity. We shall examine its effectiveness in later chapters.

---

* The MRC Biostatistics Unit estimate covers England. Up to 21 May 2021, the estimated **attack rate** (the proportion infected) was 19% (19%–20%). This model estimate is subject to revision.

Disease and Illness

How ill do people get with Covid-19?

It is a myth that statisticians love averages.* While a single summary number is important, the variability around that central figure reflects the full diversity of experience. The human reaction to viral infection shows great variety – some may not even know they have SARS-CoV-2, while others require hospitalization (see Chapter 9).

What symptoms do people experience?

Many studies have reported the symptoms experienced in cases confirmed by a PCR test, but these analyses suffer a major flaw: such symptoms are likely to have led to the person getting tested in the first place, and so these cases are not representative of all infections. To avoid potential biases we ideally need a random sample of all those carrying an infection.

Again, the ONS Covid-19 Infection Survey provides some appropriate data.[1] Participants were asked whether they were experiencing the symptoms shown in Figure 8–1, and then were given a PCR test. Only 'strong-positive' cases were used (Ct less than 30), to exclude those at the start or end of the infection.

---

* As the writer and broadcaster Timandra Harkness has said: 'Why should you never call a statistician "average?" Because it's mean.'

The most common symptoms were fatigue, coughs, and headaches

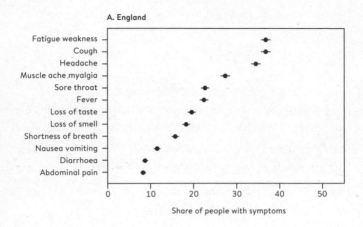

A. England

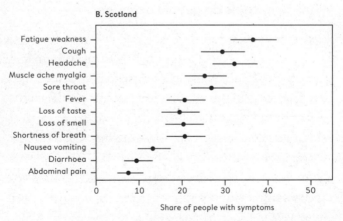

B. Scotland

Figure 8–1

Proportions of people with 'higher-evidence' positive tests (Ct less than 30) who reported each symptom, given in order of frequency, in UK nations between December 2020 and April 2021.

Source: Office for National Statistics – Covid-19 infection survey

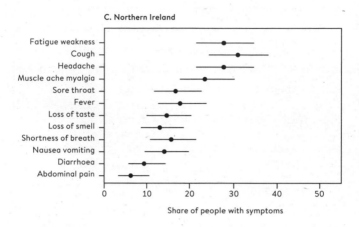

C. Northern Ireland

Share of people with symptoms

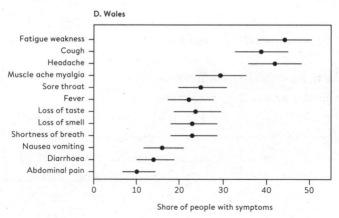

D. Wales

Share of people with symptoms

This shows that at most 40% of people nearing peaks of infection presented any of these specific symptoms. The most common were cough, fatigue, muscle ache (myalgia) and sore throat: only around one in five said they had a loss of taste or smell. About one in two reported at least one of the established symptoms and, since experiencing symptoms instigates getting a test, that fits with the rule of thumb that less than half of infected people got a test.

How many experience 'long Covid'?

Most people with Covid-19 recover quickly. Others continue to experience debilitating symptoms for weeks or even months, a phenomenon known as 'long Covid'. Two main groups have been identified. First, there are those who have been hospitalized and continue to suffer long-term symptoms, largely explicable by the aftermath of intensive care and often with organ damage – these are examined in Chapter 9.

Second, there are those who may have had a mild infection but continue to suffer from a post-viral fatigue syndrome similar to myalgic encephalomyelitis/chronic fatigue syndrome (ME/CFS), or new or continuing Covid-19 symptoms.[2] People experience a range of conditions, such as pain, fatigue or 'brain fog', sometimes in an unpredictable manner. After being ill with Covid-19, the science writer Adam Rutherford reported breathlessness and fatigue six months later.[3]

Turning diverse experiences into data has required formal definitions:

- **acute Covid-19**: symptoms up to four weeks after confirmed infection

- **ongoing symptomatic Covid-19**: four to 12 weeks
- **post-Covid-19 syndrome**: 12 weeks or longer.

The latter two groups are generally referred to as 'long Covid'.

Great care is needed to avoid biased samples when estimating the proportion experiencing long Covid. A US preprint analysis reported that over a quarter of Covid-19 cases were experiencing symptoms two months after they were first infected, but they only looked at people engaging with health-care providers, thus biasing estimates towards more severe cases.[4]

The ONS Covid-19 Infection Survey provides a better estimate,[5] asking participants to self-report their experience. Figure 8–2 shows how the proportion with symptoms declined up to four months after documented infection, with one in seven (14%, 11%–17%) still experiencing symptoms for at least 12 weeks. There were slightly higher rates in women than men, with the highest in those aged 35–69 – this is not primarily a condition of the young. These were not only the normal symptoms we all occasionally experience: the control group of people unlikely to have had Covid-19 reported a rate of about 2%.

The main persistent symptoms for 12 weeks were the same as those experienced at five weeks: fatigue (8%), headache (7%), cough (7%) and muscle ache (6%). The response options did not include 'brain fog'.

When it came to managing such long-term effects, a group of experts concluded there was no good-quality published evidence on effective interventions, and the panel 'largely based its recommendations on its own clinical and lived experience'.[6]

The share reporting symptoms after Covid-19 was higher than for control participants

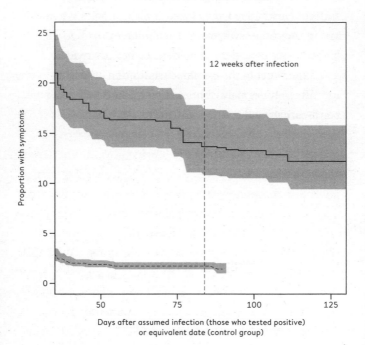

Figure 8–2
Estimated percentage of people who reported any symptom following confirmed Covid-19 infection in the UK from April 2020 to March 2021 – the symptoms elicited are those in Figure 8-1. The bands show 95% confidence intervals.

- - - - Control
———— Participants who tested positive for Covid-19

Source: Office for National Statistics – Coronavirus (Covid-19) Infection Survey

This is a virus which produces a huge variety of responses, and scientists are still seeking to understand biological mechanisms behind continued harm. The ONS survey estimated that about 1.1 million people (one in 60 of the population) were suffering from long Covid in April 2021, including 'brain fog' and various other symptoms. That is likely to reduce quality of life and place considerable burdens on health services.

As the worst of the epidemic passes, and most of us return to reasonably normal activities, it will be important to remember those facing the long-term impacts of infection.

What happened in hospitals?

After SARS-CoV-2 invades your body, the virus hijacks cells,[1] turning them into viral factories which go on to infect other cells. The immune system responds, but can cause inflammation in the lungs, leading to breathing difficulties. The body lacks oxygen, inducing widespread distress. SARS-CoV-2 can also attack other organs, including the heart, blood vessels and brain. Harlan Krumholz, a cardiologist at Yale University, said the disease 'can attack almost anything in the body with devastating consequences'.[2] The understanding of how Covid-19 affects the human body is growing.

Given its ease of spread and severity, this disease puts great pressure on hospitals.

How many people have gone to hospital with Covid-19?

In Italy on 12 March 2020, there were around 8,000 hospital patients with Covid-19, mainly clustered in a single region. A nurse likened the coronavirus outbreak 'to a world war'.[3] The national hospitalized number reached about 33,000 on 4 April.

Figure 9–1 shows weekly admissions per 100,000 people for four countries. In the week ending 22 March 2020,[4] Italy reported about 30 Covid-19 hospital admissions per 100,000,

In these four countries, weekly Covid-19 admissions rose in the winter of 2020

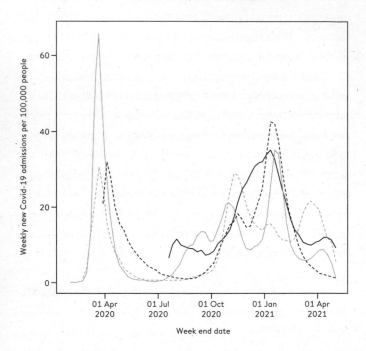

Figure 9–1

Weekly new Covid-19 admissions per 100,000 people between March 2020 and April 2021 for Italy, Spain, the UK and US.

——— United States   ——— Spain

- - - - Italy   - - - - - United Kingdom

Source: Our World in Data, using ECDC for EU countries and government sources elsewhere

while Spain reported 66.[5] The UK's weekly peak of 42 Covid-19 admissions per 100,000 came during the second wave in the week ending 10 January 2021.

Under normal conditions, English hospitals admitted around 600 patients a week per 100,000 people in 2018–19 and 2019–20.[6] But a highly infectious disease poses additional burdens on hospital care, out of proportion to the raw numbers.

These national averages disguise larger local peaks. London reached a peak of 52 Covid-19 admissions per 100,000 people in the first week of 2021:[7] about one in every 1,920 Londoners was admitted. Queues of ambulances built up, and the Mayor of London, Sadiq Khan, declared a 'major incident': 'the situation in London is now critical with the spread of the virus out of control'.[8] At that time, every region in the UK saw admission rates of more than 19 per 100,000. In total, up to 31 March 2021 there were about 458,000 Covid-19 hospital admissions in the UK* – nearly half a million.

How did the NHS cope?

Right from the start of the pandemic, the fear was that the NHS would be overwhelmed, normal care would disintegrate and staff and patients would suffer unduly; this led to the government's slogan 'Stay Home, Protect the NHS, Save Lives'. Fortunately, the NHS did not collapse, but it was subjected to massive pressure which was inadequately reflected in statistics.

---

* In England and Scotland, a Covid-19 admission is counted if the person tested positive in the previous 14 days. Northern Ireland counts 'confirmed' Covid-19 admissions with a specific method of admission codes. Unlike the other nations, Wales also includes suspected patients with Covid-19 in their overall count. For patients who get a positive test while in hospital, the 'admission date' is the day before diagnosis.

Staff absences rose from the normal 4% to over 6% in April 2020, due both to illness with Covid-19 and to self-isolation. That is equivalent to nearly 80,000 full-time staff being absent each month – enough for ten large hospitals.[9] If we consider just absences put down to infectious diseases, that month nearly a million working days were lost, forty times the past average.

Despite huge efforts, normal NHS service was seriously disrupted. In England[10] there were about 4.4 million people on waiting lists for treatment in February 2020, a figure that had been steadily increasing for years.[11] By April 2021 the number exceeded 5 million for the first time. During the first wave nearly 90,000 joint-replacement surgeries were cancelled,[12] leaving many struggling with daily pain.

Seven new Nightingale hospitals were rapidly put together, but hardly used, partly because referring hospitals were unable to spare accompanying staff. The 4,000-bed facility at London's ExCeL centre reportedly treated 54 patients in the first wave.[13] The total cost of these now-closed hospitals was over £500 million.[14]

What happened to people in hospital with Covid-19?

Covid-19 was a new disease; initially it had no specific treatments. Doctors were left healing manifest symptoms. Most Covid-19 patients were treated on the wards, although severe cases could be admitted to critical care (intensive-care or high-dependency units), usually within 24 hours of admission.

As we shall see in Chapter 10, clinicians learned from each other, testing treatments and improving care. As pressure eased in the first wave, there was a profound reduction in death rates; in-hospital mortality within 28 days of admission fell from 30–35% in early March and April 2020[15] to 10–15% for admissions in late July and August that year. In the second wave,[16] hospital mortality was around 20%.*

Figure 9–2 shows a rough estimate of what happened to 100 admissions in the first wave. As we saw in Chapter 1, those who go into critical care tend to be younger than those admitted to hospital wards, selected as best able to withstand and benefit from the rigours of treatment. Many older patients with extensive co-morbidities remain on the wards.

The reports from the Intensive Care and National Audit and Research Centre (ICNARC) cover over 24,000 critical-care admissions from 1 September 2020 to 25 March 2021.[17] ICNARC described an excess of patients with Asian and Black ethnicity (21%) and from deprived communities. Also, 12% of these patients had a BMI of 40 or more ('severely obese'), compared to about 3% of all English adults.[18] Males outnumbered females by two to one.

ICNARC reported an overall mortality rate in critical care of around 37%, but varying hugely by age. About 66% of critical-care patients aged 80 or over died within 28 days, compared to 12% of those aged 16–39. Men had a higher likelihood of death than women, but deprivation or ethnicity appeared to have little extra effect on the mortality risk.

The poet Michael Rosen, the Children's Laureate from

---

* Between 1 August 2020 and 31 March 2020, NHS England reported around 282,000 Covid-19 admissions and 57,000 Covid-19 hospital deaths within 28 days of a positive test.

This is what happened to a cohort of Covid hospital patients in the first wave

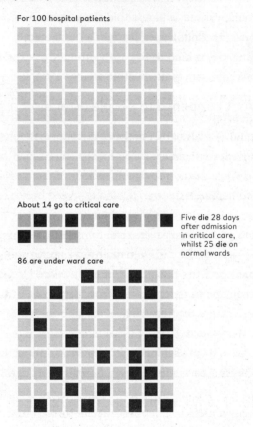

For 100 hospital patients

About 14 go to critical care

Five **die** 28 days after admission in critical care, whilst 25 **die** on normal wards

86 are under ward care

Figure 9–2
Outcomes for the ISARIC WHO CCP-UK cohort of 63,972 patients in Great Britain admitted between 9 March and 2 August 2020, scaled to 100. Critical care has a higher proportion of deaths, but most hospital deaths occurred in standard care.

Source: Changes in hospital mortality in the first wave of Covid-19 in the UK using the ISARIC WHO Clinical Characterisation Protocol: prospective observational cohort study

2007 to 2009, was in his 70s when he was admitted to critical care with Covid-19. He later recalled being asked to give informed consent for mechanical ventilation; Rosen asked if he would wake up and was told there was a 50–50 chance if he consented, but zero if he didn't.[19] The doctors were, if anything, being kind to him: of ventilated over-70s in the first wave, about 70% died within 28 days.

What happened to people after discharge?

An ONS analysis[20] of hospital discharges in England up to 31 August 2020 showed that those treated for Covid-19 fared far worse than other patients. Of each 100 Covid-19 patients who had been discharged and followed up for an average of 4–5 months, 29 had been readmitted to hospital and 12 had died, much higher rates than for non-Covid-19 patients.

An analysis of US Veteran Affairs health-care-system hospitals came to similar conclusions.[21] Of the 1,775 veterans with Covid-19 discharged between 1 March and 1 July 2020, 354 (20%) were readmitted and 162 (9%) died within 60 days of leaving hospital.

Severe Covid-19, and its treatment, causes morbidity as well as death. Leaving the hospital is not the end of the problem.

How many caught Covid-19 in hospital?

An outbreak of Covid-19 in hospital can have devastating effects. A single unsuspected case in St Augustine's Hospital in South Africa led to six major clusters,[22] resulting in confirmed infections among 80 members of staff and 39 patients, 15 of whom died.

It is difficult to find accurate data on hospital-acquired

infections of SARS-CoV-2. NHS England advised Full Fact, a fact-checking organization, to calculate 'probable nosocomial infections'[23] – those originating in hospital – by subtracting 'new hospital cases from the community' (confirmed at or soon after admission) from 'new hospital cases' (confirmed at any point in their stay). Using this method, between 1 August 2020 and 31 March 2021 there were around 40,900 probable infections in hospital. That means about one in seven new hospital cases first tested positive at least a week after admission.

According to the *Guardian*, 'NHS England insisted that the real rate of hospital-acquired coronavirus is 4.5%.'[24] That figure uses a different definition: in-patient diagnoses with first specimen dates at least 14 days after admission, which could be considered a 'definite' in-hospital infection.

Figure 9–3 shows that the proportion of probable hospital-acquired SARS-CoV-2 infections had a distinct trend, rising to over one in five during the winter peak.

This discussion of Covid-19 in hospitals cannot adequately reflect the suffering experienced by patients – particularly with restrictions on family visits – and hospital staff, working long shifts in incredibly challenging conditions while trying to protect their own health with intrusive protective equipment.

Statistics alone cannot convey these sacrifices.

In England, the share of diagnoses seven days or more after admission rose to about 1 in 4 in December 2020

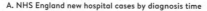

A. NHS England new hospital cases by diagnosis time

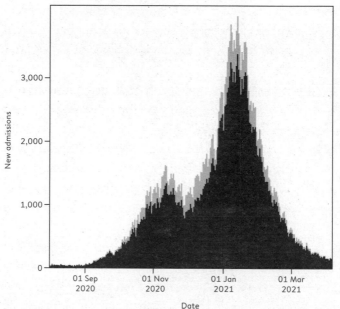

Figure 9–3

NHS England new Covid-19 hospital cases by diagnosis time and the proportion in which the first positive test was seven or more days after admission. This is for 1 August 2020–6 April 2021.

▇ Admissions or diagnoses within seven days
▨ Diagnoses after seven days

Source: NHS England: Weekly admissions and beds up to 6 April 2021

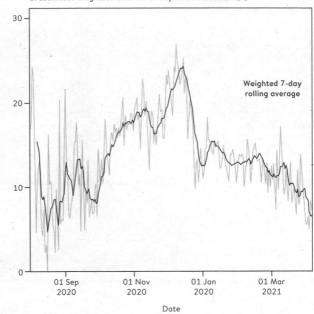

B. Estimated diagnoses after seven days from admission (%)

Weighted 7-day
rolling average

% of new admissions

Date

How good are the treatments for Covid-19?

We saw in Chapter 9 that hospital outcomes improved during the first wave, but how did this happen?

At the start of the pandemic, respiratory distress galvanized a focus on ventilators,[1] and 70% of those in critical care were invasively ventilated in the first 24 hours:[2] a tube was put down their throat and a machine took over their breathing by pushing air/oxygen into their lungs. After the downsides of 'positive-pressure' ventilation on Covid-19-infected lungs became clear, this rate dropped to around 30%. Less aggressive treatments became favoured, in which gentler air pressure is applied through a mask or other contraption with the patient remaining 'responsible' for their own respiratory effort.[3] Simple, but previously little used, interventions like getting patients to lie on their front (proning) helped them to ventilate all areas of their lungs.[4]

Many suffer serious symptoms after initial infection, needing to endure punishing treatments. An extreme case is extra-corporeal membrane oxygenation (ECMO), which requires blood to be pumped through what is essentially an 'artificial lung' by the bedside, allowing ultra-damaged lungs to rest. A national service uses points-based referral criteria, only including the sickest and excluding frail patients because of its grim effects. NHS England treated 236 patients with ECMOs in the first wave.[5] In the past, there had usually been 40 ECMO referrals a year to the Royal Papworth Hospital in Cambridge: that figure rose to 40 referrals a month.[6]

The rapid learning curve was mediated by professional grapevines, social media and online discussions of clinical practice and the latest pre-prints. But not all innovations have obvious benefits, and we need to take great care about claiming medical benefits of treatments.

As is inevitable for a new and frightening disease, we heard many claims of potentially dubious remedies. Madagascar's President Rajoelina asserted the benefits of herbal tonics,[7] while President Donald Trump gave apparent support for injecting bleach.[8] The anti-malarial drug hydroxychloroquine was heavily promoted by both the popular doctor Didier Raoult in France and Trump in the US. A paper in the prominent journal *The Lancet* appeared to confirm its benefits but had to be withdrawn when the genesis of the claimed data became suspicious.[9]

The idea of giving people blood transfusions from people who had recovered from Covid-19 (convalescent plasma) also seemed reasonable, since some immune response might be transferred. Stephen Kahn, the head of the US Food and Drug Administration, asserted a 35% reduction in mortality.*[10]

---

* Kahn's explanation was incorrect, claiming that of 100 people *ill* with Covid-19, 35 fewer would die if they received convalescent plasma. That would be remarkable, given that fewer than 35 would be expected to die anyway. What he should have said was that, of 100 *deaths* from Covid-19, 35 fewer would have happened if they had had convalescent plasma. That would turn out to be wrong too, but that was not known at the time.

All these claims were based on just comparing what happened to people who did or did not have the treatment, but this is insufficient to prove that a new treatment *caused* any differences. It may, for example, have been given to healthier patients. We could use statistical methods to adjust for known imbalances, but the main reliable way to prove causation is to allocate volunteers at random to receive the new treatment or a control. Such **randomized controlled trials** (**RCTs**) were first developed for use in agriculture, but now Web designers and analysts use randomized trials through 'A/B testing': every time you visit a website you may be taking part in multiple trials.

Randomized trials reduce statistical biases by ensuring that groups are balanced, up to the play of chance, and even in ways we are unaware could influence the outcome. If these trials are large enough, researchers can robustly say whether the intervention helped or not.

Fortunately, the UK Randomised Evaluation of Covid-19 Therapy (RECOVERY) organization[11] was set up early in the pandemic and has become the world's largest collaboration for trials on people hospitalized with Covid-19, with over 180 hospitals and about 40,000 hospital patients taking part so far. RECOVERY takes advantage of the unique NHS infrastructure to simultaneously run multiple overlapping trials, so that each patient may be in many studies. Such 'platform trials' are a recent innovation that have proved their worth.

RECOVERY trials have been hugely influential. Figure 10–1 shows the results for low-dose dexamethasone,[12] a cheap and widely used steroid. By March 2021, the use of dexamethasone was estimated to have saved 22,000 lives in the UK and over a million worldwide.[13] Another RECOVERY study showed that

Dexamethasone lowered mortality for patients needing respiratory support

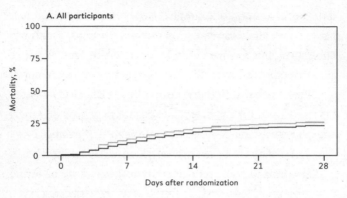

A. All participants

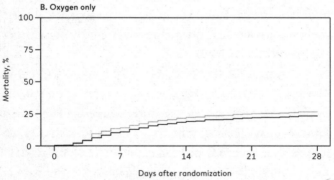

B. Oxygen only

Figure 10–1
Cumulative mortality (%) in days after randomization to either low-dose dexamethasone, an inexpensive steroid or usual care. Twenty-eight-day mortality was reduced by 27% overall but differed between patient groups. Mortality was reduced by 36% in those requiring mechanical ventilation, by 18% in those requiring oxygen only. Those not receiving oxygen did not benefit.

——— Dexamethasone   ——— Usual care

Graphical reconstruction
Source: Dexamethasone in Hospitalized Patients with Covid-19 (NEJM, 2021)

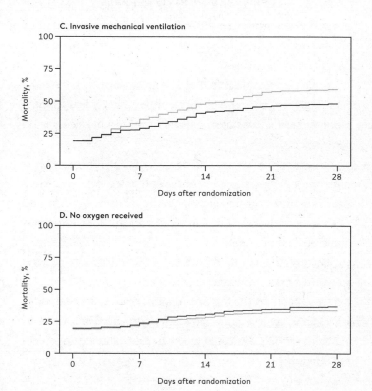

for every 25 patients treated with tocilizumab, a treatment for rheumatoid arthritis, one additional life would be saved.[14]

Randomized trials are useful for detecting small but important differences. The difference in absolute risk may not appear big, but multiplied over vast numbers of patients it means many lives saved.

Almost as valuable as finding effective treatments, RECOVERY trials also established, for example, that hydroxychloroquine did not show a clear clinical benefit,[15] and neither did convalescent plasma.[16]

Other treatments are still contested. The effects of Vitamin D as a dietary supplement are still unknown.[17] Ivermectin, a treatment for parasites in animals, has been promoted as an anti-viral treatment, but regulatory authorities recommend against its use.[18]

RECOVERY is one of the UK's greatest contributions to world health, all based on the simple principle of deciding treatments by the flip of a (digital) coin. It demonstrates what can be achieved through efficient organization, a national health service, dedicated medical teams and vast numbers of volunteers.

Deaths

How many people have died from Covid-19?

This appears a simple question to answer – we count the deaths caused by the virus. However, as we find throughout this book, the reality is somewhat more complicated. If you forgive statisticians for sounding impersonal, it is often easy to count bodies; saying whether they died because of Covid-19 is a different matter. Just in the UK there are numerous ways of tolling deaths.

What is meant by a 'death from Covid-19'?

The WHO gives the following guidance for certification of a death due to Covid-19:[1] 'a death resulting from a clinically compatible illness, in a probable or confirmed Covid-19 case, unless there is a clear alternative cause of death that cannot be related to Covid-19 disease (e.g. trauma)'. According to this wide definition there does not need to be a positive test, and Covid-19 is assumed to be the cause of death without another plausible explanation.

There are two problems with this definition. First, it depends on medical judgement about causes. Second, it can take weeks to process; it is ill suited to the demands of real-time surveillance and public appetite for rapid updates. The numbers appearing on the daily-changing dashboards draw from a parallel reporting system, separate from official death registrations.

Different counting methods complicate comparisons across countries, and even within countries. For example, the Netherlands health institute[2] publishes daily counts of Covid-19 deaths, *overleden patienten*, with a positive test, including those in care homes and other settings. Belgium's Sciensano[3] counts both confirmed and suspected Covid-19 deaths. In the US, the Centers for Disease Control and Prevention[4] includes both probable and confirmed Covid-19 deaths, depending on jurisdictions.

At the start of the pandemic NHS England was very restrictive, counting only deaths in hospital after a positive test for SARS-CoV-2. While definitions in Wales, Scotland and Northern Ireland remained constant,[5] that in England changed several times.[6] Public Health England took responsibility for this statistic on 29 April 2020,[7] expanding the definition to include deaths notified to local health protection teams. They also linked positive 'Pillar 1' test results* to death reports from electronic hospital records. That change had a dramatic effect: up to 28 April there were 19,739 reported deaths in English hospitals. The new definition increased that count by 3,811 – to 23,550 deaths.

Improved record linkage in June 2020 added more deaths. In July came a bombshell, when researchers highlighted what perhaps should have been obvious:[8] if we count everyone

---

* In the UK testing programme, Pillar 1 is swabbing those in medical need and the 'most critical key workers'.

with a positive test who subsequently dies as a Covid-19 death, then it is impossible to recover from Covid-19! An official said: 'You could have been tested positive in February, have no symptoms, then be hit by a bus in July and you'd be recorded as a Covid death.'[9]

That caused considerable consternation, with Health Secretary Matt Hancock ordering an inquiry. By 12 August, Public Health England introduced a time limit into its 'headline' number, counting any death within 28 days of a positive test for SARS-CoV-2.[10] That meant an immediate reduction in total recorded deaths by 5,377.

It's vital to remember that the daily counts on the news of the '28-day' death figures do not represent deaths that *happened* in the last 24 hours, but those newly *reported*. Figure 11–1 shows a clear weekly cycle: the daily figures tend to be higher on Tuesdays and Wednesdays because of reporting delays over the weekend. This has led to some dramatic differences in England: there were 560 deaths reported on Monday, 18 January 2021, jumping to 1,507 the next day. Since all these numbers are released at around 4 p.m. each day, they become 'news' and so are given prominence by journalists, regardless of their relevance.

The 28-day window is arbitrary; the time from test to death can be longer than four weeks, and the testing criterion

[Following pages] **Figure 11–1**
Reported deaths within 28 days of a positive test in England, for each day of the week on which they are reported. There are very different patterns according to the day of the week on which deaths are reported.

Source: Public Health England Covid-19 dashboard data download

Reported deaths show a weekly cycle: Tuesday and Wednesday are higher than other days

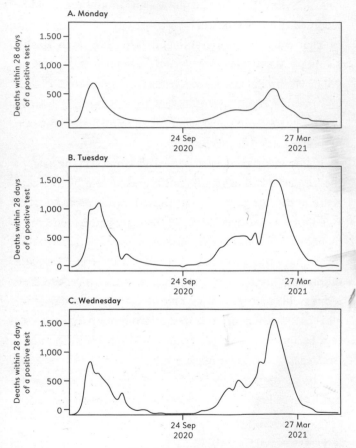

Week start date (Monday) of publication

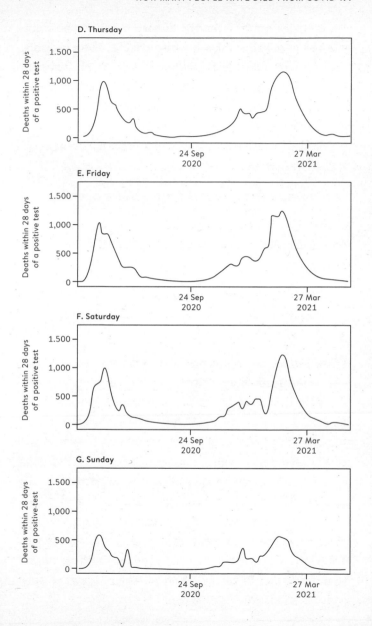

also excludes deaths from the disease of those who went untested or only had false-negative results. There is also a 60-days-'plus' count: deaths within 60 days of a positive test *or* if Covid-19 appears on the death certificate, but this could be affected even more from unrelated deaths occurring in that window.

Confused? You are not alone. And we have not even begun on death registrations.

How many 'official' deaths have there been?

As part of the death registration process, clinicians provide a medical certificate of cause of death (MCCD).[11] The MCCD has two parts:

- Part I: the sequence of disease that led to the death
- Part II: other important factors contributing to the death.

If Covid-19 appears in the first part, clinicians believe it was a cause – a death 'due to Covid-19', even if the final event before the death was, say, pneumonia. If the certificate mentions the disease in either part, it is a death 'involving Covid-19'. Unlike test-based counts, doctors do not need a positive test to believe that Covid-19 played a role in someone's death. Up to June 2020, Covid-19 was labelled as 'suspected' in 8.4% (4,251 deaths) of all deaths in which it was implicated.[12]

Figure 11–2 displays all death registrations in England and Wales between the end of 2019 and April 2021, and separates deaths with Covid-19 mentioned on the death certificate from deaths not involving Covid-19. The image generates many questions.

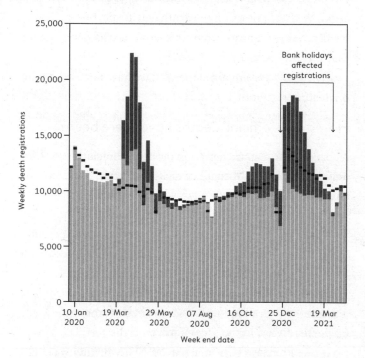

Death registrations exceeded the 2015–2019 average in two extended periods

Figure 11–2
Deaths registered in England and Wales between 28 December 2019 and 23 April 2021, by week of registration. The black line is the 2015–19 average; the dark shade indicates deaths involving Covid-19.

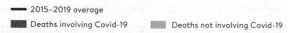

— 2015–2019 average

■ Deaths involving Covid-19   Deaths not involving Covid-19

Source: Office for National Statistics: Deaths registered weekly in England and Wales, provisional week ending 23 April 2021

During the first wave, Covid-19 deaths rose rapidly, but so did deaths from other causes. Why? The ONS has put forward possible explanations,[13] including 'collateral damage', through people avoiding overstretched hospitals. But the primary cause is likely to be under-reporting of Covid-19, especially in care homes where many people went untested, and certifying doctors might be reluctant to write Covid-19 as a cause, particularly if they had not seen the patient themselves recently. This is a novel disease: clinical judgement is challenging.

In summer 2020 Covid-19 deaths plummeted, and for a few weeks deaths from all causes were under the five-year average. The second wave saw a rise in Covid-19 deaths, as well as *deficits* of deaths not involving Covid-19, in marked contrast to the first wave. As the second wave receded, deaths from all causes decreased to low levels; in the week ending 30 April 2021 there were 9,692 deaths registered in England and Wales, 766 fewer than the five-year average and the lowest since 2014 for that week. So why were non-Covid-19 deaths so low in the second wave?

There are many potential reasons. The weather was mild. As we shall see in Chapter 17, the restrictions in place had the collateral benefits of fewer road casualties and suppressing seasonal influenza. There is no sign, yet, of increased deaths from cancer, despite disruptions to hospital services.

There is also the fact that some vulnerable people who died in the first wave might otherwise have survived another year and be dying in 2021. This **mortality displacement**, also known by the unfortunate term 'harvesting', often shows when a cluster of deaths due to extreme heat or cold is followed by a dip in mortality rates. At the start of the first wave, one of us (DS) was quoted as saying, 'many people who die of Covid would have died anyway within a short period'. Others estimated that this proportion could be over half. We were wrong: it is plausible that between 5% and 15% of the 60,000 excess deaths in the first wave were hastened by under a year. The great majority of these people had their lives shortened by a somewhat greater extent; analysis suggests that, on average, around 10 years of life are lost from Covid-19 deaths in the UK,[14] and 16 years globally.[15]

Have people been dying because of Covid-19, or just with it?

Up to 28 August 2020, for most deaths (93%) where Covid-19 was mentioned on the death certificate the disease was stated as the underlying cause of mortality.[16] People were not just dying *with* Covid-19, they were dying *because* of Covid-19. That changed when the virus became rarer, with the proportion dying 'with' Covid-19 rising to 32% in late April 2021.[17] Why was this? We've seen that when the virus was less prevalent, there was a smaller proportion of 'strong' positives, and cases tended to be less severe. Those registering deaths may not have regarded Covid-19 as the underlying cause, even though the infection was present and considered to have contributed to the death in some way.

It is rare for there to be only one primary cause of death, and Covid-19 is no exception. In the first wave, in 91% of deaths involving Covid-19 there were pre-existing conditions,[18] with dementia and Alzheimer's disease present in a quarter of them. So while Covid-19 is the underlying cause of

Deaths at home continue to be above the 2015–2019 average

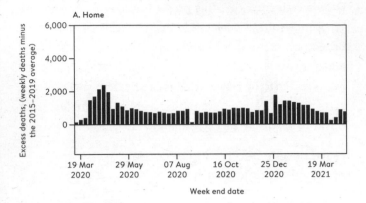

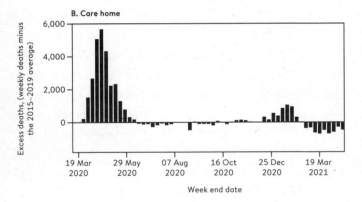

Figure 11–3

Excess deaths in England and Wales by place of death and week of death registration, from March 2020 to April 2021, compared to the 2015–19 rates for each week.

Source: Office for National Statistics: deaths registered weekly in England and Wales, provisional: week ending 23 April 2021

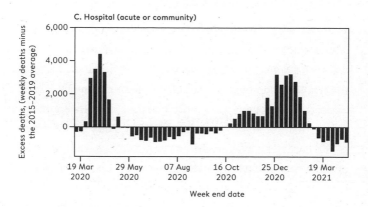

C. Hospital (acute or community)

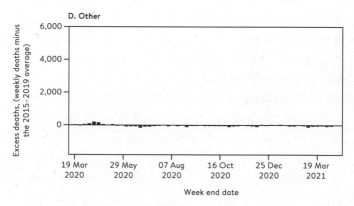

D. Other

the vast majority of Covid-19 deaths, Covid-19 is very rarely the *sole* cause.

Where have people died?

There are some striking patterns in the excess deaths for different locations, as shown in Figure 11–3 . In particular, there has been a consistent increase in deaths at home throughout the whole pandemic, at around 40%, featuring most causes of death.[19] This generates more questions: why were these people dying at home, and what was the quality of their end-of-life care? The available data cannot tell us, but putative explanations include medical advice and a personal reluctance to go to hospital unless strictly necessary. Hospitals saw surges in excess deaths in both waves, but when the pandemic waned there was a decline arising from disruption of services and the shift to dying at home.

The pattern in care homes tells a strong story; there was a massive peak of over 26,000 excess deaths in the first wave, after vulnerable care-home residents were inadequately protected.* The second wave saw few excess deaths, but this was largely because there were fewer people in care homes: residents had been removed, and those who had died had not all been replaced.

How many people have died with Covid-19?

The total toll depends on how you count. Table 11–1 summarizes three different ways of tallying the deaths in the UK,

---

* In mid-March 2020, hospitals were urged to empty wards and discharged patients were not tested, although the effect of this is contested.

Method	Total deaths: 7th March 2020 to 14th May 2021	Peak daily deaths (date of occurrence)
PHE 28-day (date of death)	127,694	1,360 (19th January 2020)
Death registrations (date of death)	153,162	1,477 (19th January 2020)
Excess deaths over five-year average	114,113	

Table 11–1
Total and peak deaths in the UK up to 14 May 2021, according to alternative methods of counting Covid-19 deaths. These provisional figures may be revised.

showing that the highest total comes from the 'official' ONS registrations. The widely reported 28-day count is timelier, but systematically undercounts Covid-19 deaths.*

Finally, the lowest total comes from excess deaths, where Covid-19 deaths may be partially countered by other deaths prevented by the measures taken.†

The apparently simple task of counting Covid-19 deaths is far from easy, with no 'true' answer. Nevertheless, however we do the counting, there is no doubt the UK has done badly.

---

* We can do the same calculations for England. Between 7 March 2020 and 14 May 2021, total deaths by occurrence date were 112,319 for the 28-day measure. For the 60-day plus measure (which is England-only), it was 130,326 – close to the death registration number of 132,023. Excess deaths by registration date over the 2015–19 average was 100,737. These are provisional figures and may be revised.

† As we shall see in Chapter 14, the total excess depends on the selected baseline.

CHAPTER 12

How lethal is SARS-CoV-2?

What are the risks of dying with Covid-19? This is an ambiguous question. We've already seen the problems of defining a 'death with Covid-19', but we must also carefully distinguish:

- The risk of both catching and dying with Covid-19, *among people who do not currently have it*. This is the **population fatality rate** (**PFR**), which will vary according to how much people have been exposed to the virus, and so depend on someone's environment and behaviour as well as how much virus there is around. It will also depend on . . .

- The risks of dying with Covid-19, *among people who get infected*. This is the **infection fatality rate** (**IFR**), which will vary according to someone's intrinsic vulnerability.*

These two measures are easily confused. As we shall see in Chapter 13, the ONS found, after adjusting for some contextual factors, that Black, Asian and minority ethnic groups were about twice as likely as people of white ethnicity to both catch

---

* There is also the case fatality rate (CFR), which is the proportion of confirmed cases that die. This is easier to observe, but confirmed cases are usually less than half of those infected.

the virus and die. But this was reported as meaning that these ethnic groups were '90% more likely to die, if they became seriously ill with Covid-19'. That was not the analytical claim and could be misleading – as we saw in Chapter 9, ethnicity does not affect the chances of surviving critical care for Covid-19.

In this chapter we will look at both types of risk for groups of different age and sex. Personalized risk factors are covered in Chapter 13.

What has been the average risk of catching the virus and subsequently dying?

The population fatality rate is the proportion of the population who die with Covid-19 over a specified period. That can be calculated from registrations of deaths 'involving Covid-19' – around 90% of these deaths will be 'from' Covid-19. Table 12–1 summarizes the experience of three disparate age groups in England and Wales, showing extraordinary differences in risk.

Out of over 7 million schoolchildren aged between five and 14, 11 died with Covid-19 mentioned on their death certificate over the year (one in 660,000). Over the same period, 469 died from other causes; Covid-19 has been a small additional risk to children, in contrast to seasonal flu, against which a vaccine is routinely offered for all children up to 12 years old.

At the other end of the scale, out of over 500,000 people aged over 90, nearly 30,000 died with Covid-19 on their death certificate (around six in 100). That is 35,000 times the risk experienced by schoolchildren. In between these extremes, about one in 730 of those aged between 55 and 64 had death involving Covid-19.

Age Group	Death involving Covid-19	2019 Population Estimate	Covid-19 rate as 1 in x	Deaths from all causes	5-year average (2015–19)	COVID-19 as % of 5-year average
5–14	11	7,257,005	1 in 660,000	480	557	2%
55–64	9,849	7,192,819	1 in 730	52,421	41,712	24%
90+	29,368	547,789	1 in 19	137,806	114,550	26%

Table 12–1
Deaths in England and Wales registered in the 52 weeks between 14 March 2020 and 12 March 2021. In this chapter, we often refer to the past averages as the 'normal' risk.

For schoolchildren, deaths involving Covid-19 represent a small share of 'normal' deaths. For both middle-aged and elderly people, the increased risk was larger and similar; it is as if all older people had their normal risk of death increased by about 25% – in effect they experienced 15 months of risk, rather than a year. This common **relative risk** will have a much bigger impact on those who were at higher risk in the first place, that is the frail and elderly.

Figure 12–1 shows the population fatality rates in more detail, for both sexes and in five-year age bands. These are compared to the 'normal' death rates – the proportion of women and men in England and Wales of each age who do not reach their next birthday. Graph A has a linear scale, but this makes it difficult to see what is going on in the younger age groups. Graph B shows the same numbers on a logarithmic scale, which we introduced in Chapter 1, in which a change from one to 10 is the same size as a change from 10 to 100.

The logarithmic scale not only allows us to see the Covid-19 death rates for younger ages, but also reveals the roughly straight lines of the death rates. On the original scale, this corresponds to an exponential increase of risk with age, which means that each year of extra age increases the risk by the same relative amount – around 12% per year older, meaning that the risk of a death involving Covid-19 doubles for each six years of extra age.*

---

* This is like compound interest: a 12% increase per year over seven years leads to a total increase of $(1.12)^6$ which is around two. The line was even straighter until the vaccine roll-out in early 2021 reduced the Covid-19 mortality rate in the very elderly.

Deaths involving Covid-19 followed a similar age pattern to past death rates

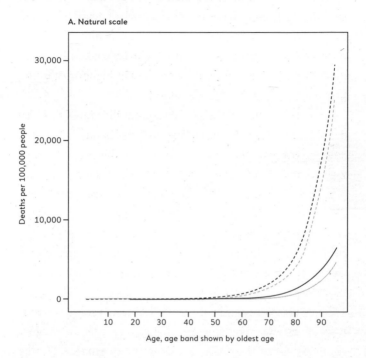

A. Natural scale

Age, age band shown by oldest age

Figure 12–1

Observed population fatality rates involving Covid-19 by age group for England and Wales registered between 14 March 2020 and 12 March 2021 (authors' calculations), compared to the average UK annual death rates for 2016–18. Rates under 0.5 are not shown.

Expected deaths by age, based on UK life tables for 2016–18	Covid-19 registrations, by age group up to 12 March 2021
----- Male ----- Female	—— Male —— Female

Authors' calculations.
Source: Office for National Statistics: UK National Life Tables, weekly death registrations (provisional) and 2019 mid-year population estimates

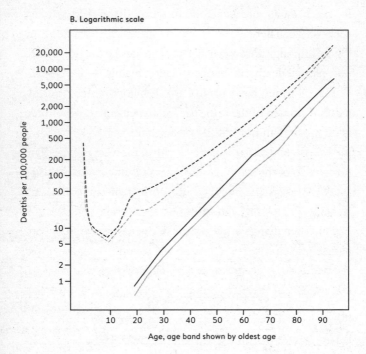

B. Logarithmic scale

Deaths per 100,000 people

Age, age band shown by oldest age

The 'normal' annual death rates for children start high due to congenital diseases and birth trauma, dropping to a minimum around age nine or 10. Nobody in the history of humanity has been as safe as a contemporary first-world primary schoolchild. There is then a steady increase, apart from the 'bump' among those in their late teens and early 20s due to non-natural deaths, including suicides, mainly of young men.

Usually, men have around a 50% higher annual mortality than women of the same age, but Covid-19 punishes men even more than normal life does: there is about 70% additional risk of death involving Covid-19 for men over 40 than for women of the same age, although it is unclear why this is.

For over-45s, the Covid-19 and 'normal' mortality lines are roughly parallel. This indicates that the average risk of catching and then dying with the virus in the first year of the pandemic was in proportion to the background risk. As we noted above, for those aged over 45, Covid-19 represented about an extra 25% over the background risk.*

What is the average risk of dying, for people who get infected with Covid-19?

This is the infection fatality rate (IFR). The overall global average IFR has been contested, with early estimates ranging from less than 0.1% (one dying in 1,000 people infected), which would make it like seasonal flu, to over 1% (one in 100). Analysis of around 200,000 Covid-19 deaths from the

---

* Since the average risk of death normally increases by about 10% for each year we get older, it is as if we were all effectively around two to three years older during the pandemic year.

first wave in 10 countries[2] showed that the risk varied enormously according to age. The average IFR might be 0.23% in a typical low-income country with a young population, and 1.15% in a typical high-income country such as the UK.* It is far worse than flu.†

Figure 12–2 shows deaths per 100,000 people infected for different ages (in circles), compared to the average annual mortality rate from all causes between 2016 and 2018.

The lines are remarkably similar, giving a simple interpretation: on average, being infected with SARS-CoV-2 contributes about a year's worth of extra lethal risk, thus doubling the risk that people already face of not reaching their next birthday, whatever their age.‡ This interpretation refers to averages over populations. In Chapter 13 we find other factors influencing individual risk, although there is close agreement between the factors impacting on death from Covid-19 and those for death from other causes.[3] The virus seems to pick on and amplify underlying vulnerabilities.

On a more technical point, all quoted risks are the average

---

* These are the IFR estimates without **seroreversion** (assuming antibodies do not wane over time). With seroreversion, the two estimates are 0.22% and 1.06% respectively.

† One prominent critic of lockdowns claimed in a (subsequently deleted) Tweet that the infection fatality rate was 0.1%, as 5 million people had been infected and 50,000 had died. Unfortunately, some simple arithmetic reveals that this means the IFR is 1%, not 0.1%.

‡ Unfortunately, the message that Covid-19 risk was about the same as the annual risk has been misinterpreted as meaning that infection does not increase the annual risk at all. That misunderstanding led to a May 2020 online newspaper headline that read 'CALMING FEARS: Your risk of dying is NO different this year – despite coronavirus pandemic, says expert'. DS was that expert, and got the headline changed.

Additional estimated mortality from infection is similar to the average past mortality rates

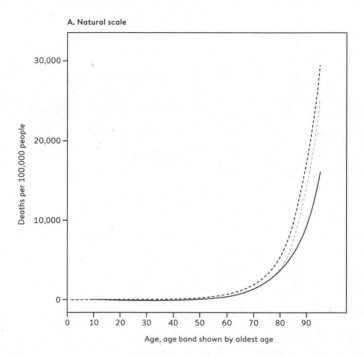

A. Natural scale

Deaths per 100,000 people

Age, age band shown by oldest age

Figure 12-2

Age-specific mortality rates per 100,000 following infections estimated in October 2020, compared with actuarial proportion of women and men dying each year of any cause (based on 2016–18 England and Wales life tables).

Expected deaths by age, based on UK life tables for 2016–18

- - - - - Male   - - - - - Female   ———— Estimated additional mortality if infected

Source: Office for National Statistics: UK National Life Tables, Imperial College London: Report 34 – Covid-19 Infection Fatality Ratio Estimates from Seroprevalence

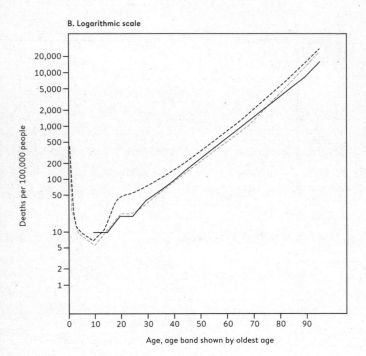

B. Logarithmic scale

Deaths per 100,000 people

Age, age band shown by oldest age

(mean) for people of those ages. These are not the risks of the 'average person', as much of the population's mortality risk is covered by those who are already ill – the distribution of risk is highly skewed. For most healthy people, the risk of dying from Covid-19 or anything else is much lower than that stated here.

With lower viral prevalence and greater vaccine protection, the future risk of getting Covid-19 and dying should be different from that described in this chapter. The fatality rate of infected people may also reduce over time, with milder forms of the disease and improving treatments.

We can hope that vulnerable people will not be exposed to such high risks again.

CHAPTER 13

Who has been most at risk from Covid-19?

We have already seen the importance of age and sex in determining the risks from Covid-19, but attention has also focused on factors such as ethnicity, deprivation, occupation and medical conditions. These are often strongly related, and so it is hard to separate their effects. A further challenge is that looking at Covid-19 death rates in different groups does not tell us whether they are at higher risk of infection or have worse outcomes after catching the virus.

How has ethnicity affected the risk of dying from Covid-19?

When we analyse what has happened to people of different ethnicity, we are looking at a complex web of culture, religion, lifestyle, family, housing, employment, health and more. The ONS tried to disentangle some of these influences, which involved complex linking of different datasets, as ethnicity is not mentioned on death certificates.

Figure 13–1 looks at the link between ethnicity and deaths involving Covid-19 during the first wave,[1] first adjusting for the different age profile of ethnic groups and then for other factors.

Relative to the white population, age-adjusted death rates

There are heightened rates of Covid-19 deaths in English ethnic minorites

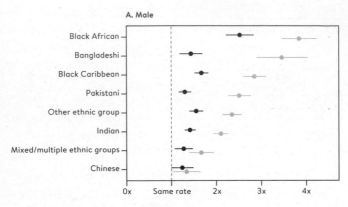

A. Male

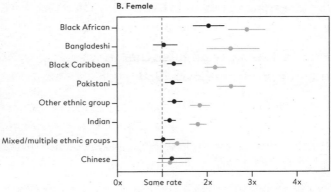

B. Female

Hazard ratio, rates of death involving
Covid-19 relative to white people

were higher for all ethnic groups: the death rate among Black Africans was nearly four times higher for men and three times higher for women. After adjusting for geography, deprivation and pre-existing medical factors, the death rates for most ethnic groups came closer to white people. That suggests increased risks were not genetic, but more associated with living circumstances and factors such as occupation and access to health care.

In the second wave[2] the effects arising from Black ethnicity fell, while those linked to Bangladeshi and Pakistani ethnicity rose. It is unclear why.

Could these findings be primarily due to increased risks of infection? Before the vaccination programme, a REACT-2 study[3] showed, after adjustment for age, sex and region, that people of Asian ethnicity had a 56% (39%–75%) higher rate of antibodies than those of white ethnicity, while the estimated rate in Black communities was more than double. There are many reasons why some ethnic-minority groups had higher rates of Covid-19 infection, linked to higher rates of at-risk occupations, more deprivation and multi-generational households. In January–March 2019, 24% and 16% people

[Facing page] Figure 13–1
Rates of death involving Covid-19 by ethnic group and sex, relative to white people, for deaths in England between 2 March 2020 and 28 July 2020. Horizontal bars show 95% confidence intervals around the estimates. 'Adjusting for' means attempting to eliminate the impact of place of residence, different levels of deprivation and health status. This will not be perfect.

Adjusted for ● Age   ● Age, geography, socio-economics, and health status

Source: Office for National Statistics – Explaining ethnic background contrasts in deaths involving Coronavirus (Covid-19)

of Bangladeshi and Black African backgrounds respectively lived in overcrowded housing, compared with 2% of those from a white British background.[4]

An OpenSAFELY study found there were similar ethnic differences both for testing positive and for dying with Covid-19, which 'suggests that ethnic differences in death might be mediated through exposure or susceptibility to infection, rather than through susceptibility to severe disease once infected'.[5] The way in which communities engage with the health-care system is also likely to play a role.

How have occupations affected Covid-19 risks?

Certain public-facing jobs have greater exposure to infection, which can feed into death rates. Figure 13–2 shows an ONS analysis covering 2020, demonstrating substantial differences between occupations.[6] Similarly to normal life, professionals have much lower mortality risk and manual workers higher risk, although these official occupational groupings are far from homogenous.

The ONS also gives more granular occupational groups. Some stand out and can be compared with the broad groupings in Figure 13–2: of men, 82 chefs died (age-standardized mortality of 103 per 100,000), 209 taxi and cab drivers and chauffeurs (101 per 100,000), and 83 bus and coach drivers (70 per 100,000).

Among social-care workers there were 469 deaths involving Covid-19: around twice the population average for both men and women. The pattern differed for health-care workers: men had a higher mortality rate than average (190

Men and women in elementary and caring occupations had the highest Covid-19 death rates

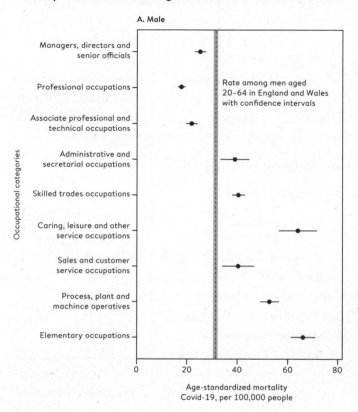

Figure 13–2

Male and female age-standardized mortality rates for Covid-19 (with 95% uncertainty intervals), for people aged 20 and 64. Data for England and Wales, between 9 March and 28 December 2020, compared to the national average for men and women. The official major occupational groups are shown: 'elementary occupations' means simple routine tasks not requiring educational qualifications.

Source: Office for National Statistics – Deaths registered in England and Wales

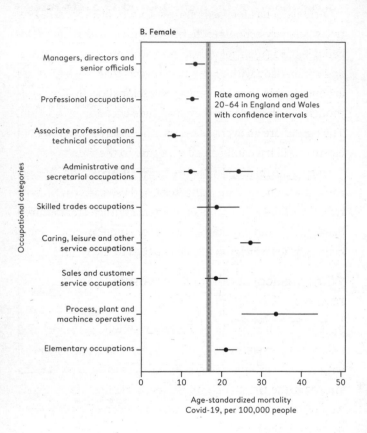

B. Female

Rate among women aged 20–64 in England and Wales with confidence intervals

Occupational categories

- Managers, directors and senior officials
- Professional occupations
- Associate professional and technical occupations
- Administrative and secretarial occupations
- Skilled trades occupations
- Caring, leisure and other service occupations
- Sales and customer service occupations
- Process, plant and machince operatives
- Elementary occupations

0   10   20   30   40   50

Age-standardized mortality
Covid-19, per 100,000 people

deaths – 45 per 100,000), while that of women was similar to the population average.

Attention has focused on risks to schoolteachers. Fifty-two secondary-school teachers died with Covid-19 up to December 2020 (men 39 per 100,000; women 21 per 100,000), and comparison with Figure 13–2 reveals that these rates are around double those in other professional occupations, although the absolute numbers preclude accurate estimation. The figures are an average across nine months, when school closures will have influenced exposure to the virus.

Just as the relationship between Covid-19 risk and age mirrored that in normal life (Chapter 12), these patterns broadly reflect the pre-Covid-19 major differences in age-standardized death rates from all causes, except for some specific public-facing groups which were more exposed to the virus.

What medical conditions increase risks from Covid-19?

Back in March 2020,[7] over 2 million people in the UK were labelled as clinically extremely vulnerable and told to shield, with specific groups being selected according to what was known at the time. High mortality in the first wave means we now have a better idea of who has been at most risk of dying from the virus.

Figure 13–3 shows an analysis by the OpenSAFELY team of factors associated with nearly 11,000 deaths with Covid-19 in the first wave, based on over 17 million medical records from GPs.[8] The influence of occupation cannot be assessed in this model as it is not included in the medical records.

The first impression is the huge effect of age. As we saw in

In the OpenSAFELY model, age dominates other factors for Covid-19 related deaths

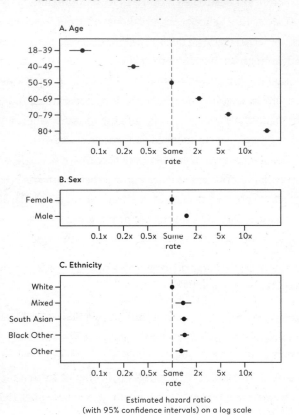

Estimated hazard ratio
(with 95% confidence intervals) on a log scale

Figure 13–3

The relative risk of both catching and dying from the virus associated with a range of clinical factors,* for English patients between February and May 2020. These are adjusted for all the other factors, attempting to estimate the size of the association while keeping everything else fixed.

Source: Nature: Factors associated with Covid-19-related death using OpenSAFELY

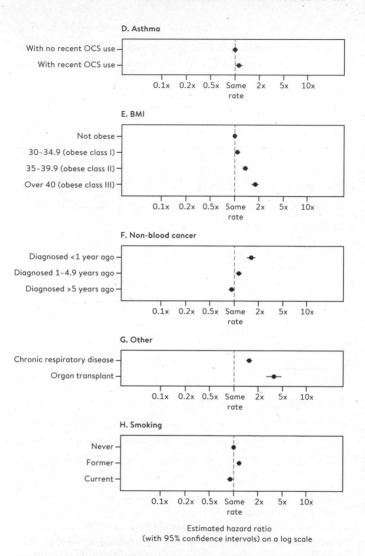

Estimated hazard ratio
(with 95% confidence intervals) on a log scale

---

* These are expressed as **hazard ratios**: the relative risks over a short period
of time, relative to a baseline category which has a hazard ratio of one. If no
baseline category is shown, it is simply the absence of the condition.

Chapter 12, each 10-year increase more than doubles the risk; this virus, just like normal life, persecutes older people. The overall effect of non-white ethnicity, after adjusting for age and medical conditions, is less than that of being 10 years older.*

Figure 13–3 allows us to see roughly how medical conditions might translate to additional years of 'effective age'. For example, an organ transplant roughly multiplies the risk by four, equivalent to being around 15 years older. The ALAMA system uses this idea by translating all medical conditions into their effect on your 'Covid-19 age', and their detailed tables permit a refined estimate of individual vulnerability.[9] This has been useful for occupational health advice.

Most medical risk factors, while important, are of limited impact compared with older age. We shall see in Chapter 24 how this affected the choice of vaccination priorities.

How did data influence shielding?

Data collected in the first wave allowed a reappraisal of the initial shielding recommendations. QCovid,[10] a system based on 6 million GP records, provided an estimate of personalized risk in the first wave, and its first results led, for example, to Down's syndrome being added to the clinically vulnerable list. In February 2021,[11] the shielded list was

---

* Scrutiny reveals one odd aspect of Figure 13–3: the apparent *protective* effect of being a current smoker. This has been a consistent observation in multiple studies and provoked considerable controversy. One possibility is that by controlling for factors that are influenced by smoking, we may be distorting any causal relationship between smoking and Covid-19 risk; in statistical terms, this is known as **collider bias**. A model that only adjusts for demographic factors (age, sex, deprivation and ethnicity) showed a positive link between smoking and death from Covid-19.

further supplemented with those QCovid considered higher-risk.*[12] Nobody was removed from the shielding list, even if they did not meet these criteria; perhaps it was felt that people might have found it hard to accept they had been shielding for nearly a year when their risk was not considered high.

We saw in Chapter 12 how Covid-19 multiplied the average risks people of different ages faced in pre-Covid-19 times. Further analysis has confirmed this idea at a more personal level:[13] the factors that were linked to Covid-19 deaths were broadly the same as those for non-Covid-19 deaths, although older age, male sex, deprivation and obesity had a stronger link with Covid-19 mortality.†

The recurrent picture is that Covid-19 multiplies any pre-existing risk by roughly the same amount for everyone. This common *relative risk* has little impact on healthy younger people, but has a major impact on the older and more vulnerable.

This virus is a bully.

---

* This included people whose absolute risk of a first-wave Covid-19 death was estimated to be more than 0.5% (one in 200), *or* had a risk greater than 10 times that of a healthy person of the same age and sex. If shielding were based solely on absolute risk – dominated by age – then many healthy older people would be included. Without the relative risk criterion, younger people with serious medical conditions would be absent.

† DS was a member of the team that carried out this comparison of over 17,000 Covid-19 and 134,000 non-Covid-19 deaths in 2020. All non-white ethnic groups had higher relative risks than white ones of Covid-19 death but, perhaps surprisingly, lower relative risk of non-Covid-19 death.

How do we compare countries?

There have been many claims about why some countries have fared better or worse than others. Such comparisons are fraught with challenges, as countries have different population structures, health policies, climate, social administrations and cultures. Countries also count things differently: some include 'probable' Covid-19 deaths; others only report lab-confirmed figures, or confirmed deaths within hospitals, or within time limits. Creating macabre league tables is overprecise; this is not the Eurovision Song Contest.

One solution is to ignore what countries call a 'Covid-19 death' and instead look at **all-cause mortality**. Such comparisons can only be made among countries that maintain accurate death registrations, which is not always the case. We can then calculate **excess deaths**[1] over a baseline value chosen to represent a 'normal' number of deaths. Excess mortality can help try to answer the crucial, counterfactual question: how does the number of deaths during the Covid-19 pandemic differ to what might have happened anyway? Statisticians also try to calculate those figures in a consistent way across countries.

Excess mortality can be hard to interpret. Changes in deaths might be due to the virus, or critical care being overwhelmed, or disruption to health services, or the impact of anti-virus measures.[2] All of these get combined into an overall count.

What 'baseline' should we use?

There is no 'correct' way of calculating excess deaths. As we saw in Chapter 11, regular reporting of death registrations for England and Wales compares deaths in the latest week to the average number of deaths over the previous five years. Other agencies use baselines accounting for trends[3] or 'normal' winters,[4] but reach similar conclusions.

There is a wide variety of reporting practices for Covid-19 deaths in different jurisdictions in the US, and so the analysis of excess deaths by the Centers for Disease Control and Prevention (CDC) becomes even more important. This is shown in Figure 14–1.

Figure 14–1 shows that excess mortality in the US peaked in April and December 2020, with a smaller peak in July–August. It never dropped to 'normal' in the summer, as occurred in the UK, but did so by March 2021. For 2020, the CDC estimated 457,000–531,000 excess deaths, compared to around 352,000 reported Covid-19 deaths.

How should we compare deaths from all causes between countries?

Comparing total number of excess deaths would unfairly penalize larger countries. A better way is to look at the increase in excess deaths relative to the baseline, where for example an increase of 100% represents a doubling.

Table 14–1 shows an analysis by Ariel Karlinsky and Dmitry

Once US death numbers elevated, they did not return to the past range in 2020

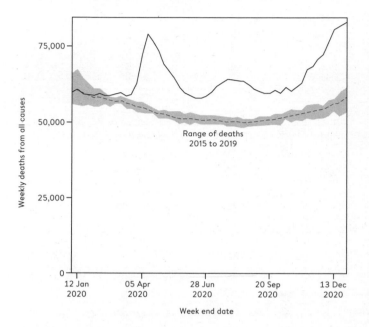

Figure 14–1

Weekly all-cause mortality in the US in 2020, compared to average and range over previous five years; as there is a lag between death and reporting, the CDC produces a 'predicted' time series.[5]

——— Deaths in 2020   – – – – Average of deaths 2015 to 2019

Source: Our World in Data (using CDC estimates): Excess mortality during the Coronavirus pandemic (Covid-19)

Country	Data up to	Reported Covid-19 deaths	Estimated excess deaths	Ratio of excess to reported Covid-19 deaths	Excess per 100,000 population	Excess relative change over baseline
Bolivia	31 January 2021	10,000	29,000	2.8	260	55%
Ecuador	28 March 2021	17,000	48,000	2.9	280	62%
Mexico	14 February 2021	170,000	400,000	2.3	320	52%
New Zealand	14 March 2021	26	–1,900		–40	–6%
Peru	4 April 2021	53,000	140,000	2.7	450	114%
Russia	28 February 2021	85,000	440,000	5.2	300	25%
United Kingdom	14 March 2021	130,000	120,000	1.0	180	20%
United States	21 February 2021	500,000	580,000	1.2	180	20%

Table 14–1
For selected countries, rounded numbers of reported Covid-19 deaths and excess mortality, the ratio, excess deaths per 100,000 people and the relative change. The values are rounded, so the relationship between columns is not exact.

Kobak comparing excess deaths versus modelled expected deaths.[6] Their analysis found that the pandemic exacted a high toll, with some countries apparently substantially under-reporting Covid-19 deaths, and Peru more than doubling its usual mortality rate.* In contrast, New Zealand showed a deficit in deaths, largely due to a reduction in flu during the winter.

Many reports also look at deaths per million people, but this does not allow for different age structures.[7] In Italy, about 23% of the population are above 65 years of age, compared to 18% in the UK and 14% in Ireland, and so a virus attacking older people would result in more deaths in Italy than in Ireland, even with the same 'performance'. This leads naturally to using an **age-standardized mortality rate**, in which the mortality rates in each age group are weighted according to a standard population.[8]

Figure 14–2 shows an analysis of age-standardized mortality in 2020,† weighted to a '2013 European Standard

---

* In June 2021, Peru revised its official Covid-19 death toll to bring it more in line with excess deaths.

† This is a complex behind-the-scenes analysis: for most European countries in the dataset, the figures are by date of death rather than date of registration, and there are also misalignments in terms of when weeks start and end.

[Following pages] Figure 14–2
Age-standardized excess deaths as a percentage of five-year average in 2020. The ONS analysis uses the Eurostat database, from the week ending 3 January (week 1 of 2020) to the week ending 18 December (week 51).[10]

———— All ages ———— Under 65s

Source: Office for National Statistics – Comparisons of all-cause mortality between European countries and regions: 2020

Spain had the highest peak in relative age-standardized mortality in 2020

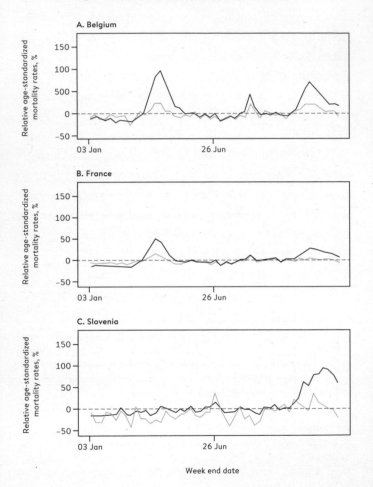

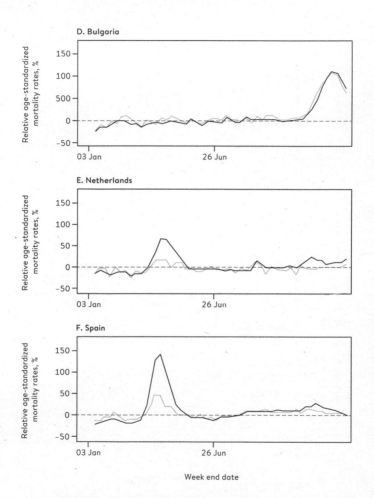

Week end date

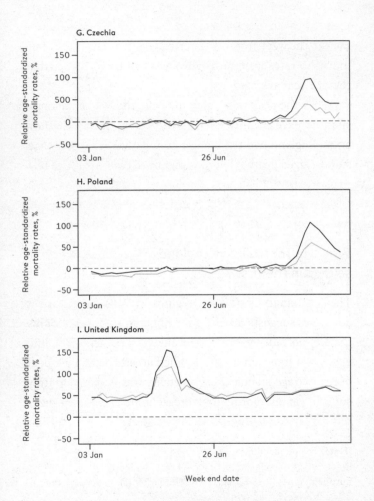

Week end date

Population' (which has 19.5% of the population over 65),[9] and expressed as a relative increase on the average over the past five years. Among 25 European countries, Spain had the highest peak in its relative age-standardized mortality rate, at 143% in the week from 28 March to 3 April 2020. That means mortality rates were nearly two and half times higher than the five-year average.

While the peak was higher in Spain, the UK had a longer span of excess mortality. By the week ending 26 June 2020, England had the highest cumulative increase in age-standardized death rates of the analysed countries. The relative increase in England was 7.5%, higher than those of Spain (5.9%), Scotland (5.3%) and Belgium (3.5%). This is a league table no one wants to head.

Why was mortality in England so high in the first wave?

The ONS analysis of small regions in Western European countries suggests a reason for England's poor outcomes. Excess mortality was more localized in countries such as Spain and Italy; among the studied areas, the highest peak of relative age-standardized mortality was Bergamo in Italy, suffering an extraordinary increase in its age-standardized rate of 842% in the week ending 20 March. The ten highest

[Following pages] Figure 14–3
Relative age-standardized mortality rates (% increase) in major European cities in 2020, from week ending 3 January (week 1 of 2020) to week ending 18 December (week 51).

——— All ages ——— Under 65s

Source: Office for National Statistics – Comparisons of all-cause mortality between European countries and regions: 2020

Madrid had the highest peak excess mortality of large cities during spring 2020

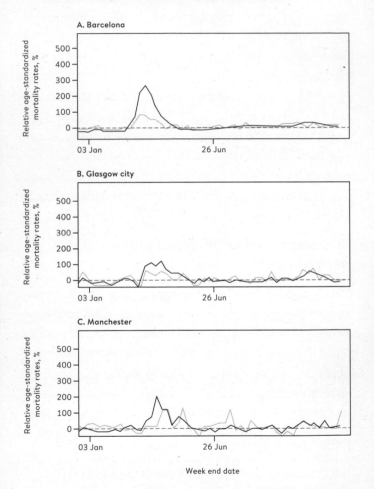

A. Barcelona

B. Glasgow city

C. Manchester

Week end date

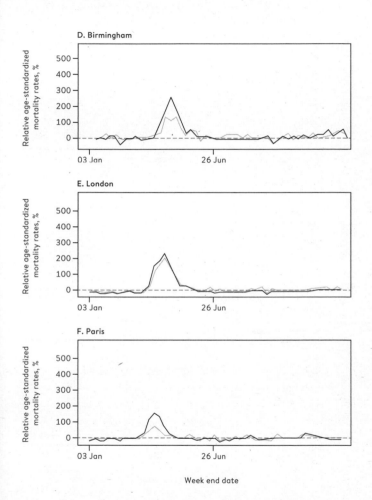

Week end date

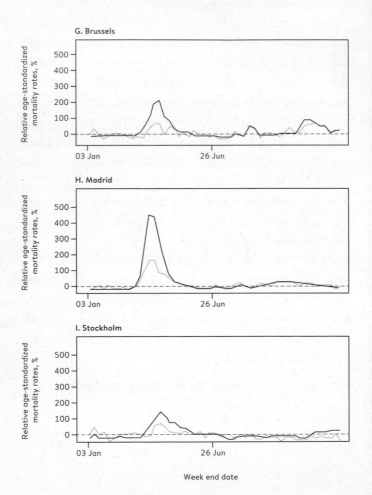

Week end date

local areas in Europe were in central Spain and northern Italy, although Figure 14–3 shows that many major European cities had similar relative excess mortality.

In contrast to these concentrated outbreaks, we saw in Chapter 2 how the virus was simultaneously introduced right across the UK. Excess deaths were therefore widespread: in the week ending 17 April 2020, of the 179 local authority areas in England 123 had a relative increase of 60% or more.

By the end of 2020, England's position in the 'league table' had dropped. Figure 14–2 shows that many eastern European countries suffered a harsh winter wave, Poland having the largest increase of the countries studied (12%). Countries such as India, which appeared to fare well initially, have since seen a surge in cases and deaths, and the picture continues to change.

In May 2020, DS wrote an article saying it would take years to assess the impact of this virus, and the picture has not changed;[11] although we can confidently conclude the UK has not done well, it is still too soon to draw any definitive conclusions.

How does the impact of Covid-19 compare with other historical harms?

There have been repeated suggestions that the harms of Covid-19 were exaggerated when compared to other threats that people largely accept.

How does Covid-19 compare with influenza?

Covid-19 and influenza are both respiratory diseases, but there are important differences. First, SARS-CoV-2 is more infectious than seasonal flu; we saw in Chapter 3 that the basic reproduction number for the original SARS-CoV-2 virus is around 3,[1] and new mutations further raised its ability to spread. By comparison, effective reproduction numbers for seasonal flu are about 1.3,[2] although they vary from year to year. In the 1918 Spanish Flu pandemic, R was higher at roughly 1.8 (1.5–2.3), but still well below the novel coronavirus. This explains why distancing and other measures, sufficient to bring R for SARS-CoV-2 to below one, are enough to almost eliminate seasonal flu.[3] That contributes to a deficit of deaths when little SARS-CoV-2 circulates.

Second, the novel virus is more deadly. As we saw in Chapter 12, the proportion of all those infected by SARS-CoV-2 who die of the disease is estimated to have been about 1.1%

in a high-income country in the first wave. The WHO states that the fatality rate of standard flu is 'usually well below 0.1%',[4] about a tenth as lethal as SARS-CoV-2.

This results in Covid-19 having greater mortal impact than seasonal flu. Flu-attributable deaths average around 10,000 each year in England,[5] but with large variation: only 4,000 in the winter of 2018–19, but over 22,000 in the preceding bad winter. These are modelled figures based on what we would expect given seasonal temperatures; on average, only about 750 death certificates a year put flu as the underlying cause of mortality between 2015 and 2019.[6]

In contrast,[7] there were about 129,000 registered deaths in England involving Covid-19 in the year from the start of the pandemic,* 90% of which had Covid-19 as the underlying cause.[8]

There is more to learn about the novel coronavirus, but it is worse than seasonal flu.

What about accidents?

Out of around 530,800 deaths registered in England and Wales in 2019, over 22,000 were 'non-natural': these included road accidents (1,502), drownings (175), accidental poisonings (3,795), suffocation (543) and a large number of falls (6,217). There were also suicides and suspected suicides (5,697) and homicides (701).[9] Life is not safe.

Since the death rates from Covid-19 change so much by age, we should compare risks for different age groups. Figure 15–1

---

* That is the number of registrations between 14 March 2020 and 12 March 2021. For registrations up to 14 May 2020, there were about 132,000 deaths involving Covid-19 in England. For the UK, the figure was 152,000.

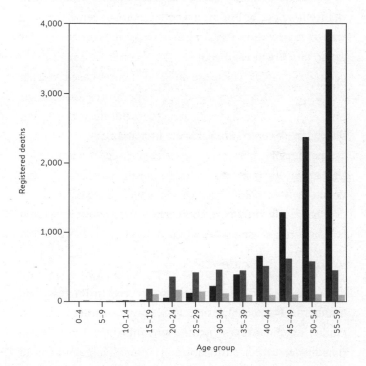

For under-60s in England and Wales, how did Covid deaths compare to normal risks?

Figure 15–1
Estimated deaths in England and Wales from injuries and accidents, road incidents (average for 2015–19) and Covid-19 (up to 12 March 2021).

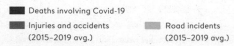

Deaths involving Covid-19

Injuries and accidents
(2015–2019 avg.)

Road incidents
(2015–2019 avg.)

Source: Office for National Statistics: (Weekly provisional death statistics and NOMIS)

shows that Covid-19 risks for younger people in the first wave were less than the ones they usually face from accidents. For each age group under 30, fewer died with Covid-19 than on average die from road accidents each year, while for each age group under 40 fewer died with Covid-19 than on average died from all accidents and injuries. Older age groups fared far worse with Covid-19.

How did deaths in 2020 compare with other years in the past?

There have been claims that the first year of Covid-19 was not particularly lethal compared to past years. Figure 15–2 (A) shows total numbers of deaths registered in England and Wales each year since 1900,[10] and we can immediately see that there are only two years when that count exceeded 600,000. These are 1918, when the Spanish Flu epidemic started, and 2020.*

The population has grown over the last 120 years, and in Figure 15–2 (B), we see the **crude mortality rate**: the number of registered deaths for every 100,000 people. As public health and treatments have improved, the rate has steadily decreased.

There was a noticeable spike in 2020, back to a level not seen since 2003. The increase from the past five-year average (in 2015–19) to 2020 is the largest since 1941, when Blitz casualties mounted. After 1900, the largest increase in crude mortality from its past five-year average was in 1918.

---

* In wartime, only deaths that occur in England and Wales are registered. Deaths abroad on active service are not included in these totals.

In 2020, there were over 608,000 death registrations in England and Wales

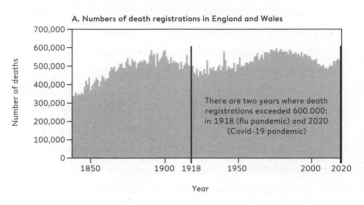

A. Numbers of death registrations in England and Wales

There are two years where death registrations exceeded 600.000: in 1918 (flu pandemic) and 2020 (Covid-19 pandemic)

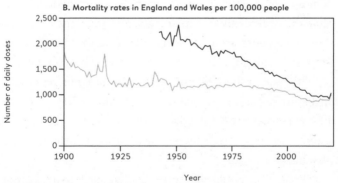

B. Mortality rates in England and Wales per 100,000 people

Figure 15–2

Graph A shows a simple count of the number of death registrations in England. Graph B shows the crude mortality rate per 100,000 people (adjusted for the size of the population), and the age-standardized mortality rate (adjusted both for the size and age structure of the population).

——— Age-standardized mortality rate ——— Crude mortality rate

Source: Office for National Statistics, 1900 to 2020 (provisional)

But the crude calculation does not account for how populations have got older, so Figure 15–2 (B) also shows the annual *age-standardized* mortality rates since 1942,* from which we can see that 2020 is not historically high. In fact, all years before 2009 had higher rates. This graph also reveals the astonishing halving of age-standardized death rates over the previous decades; life expectancy in England rose from 69 in 1950 to 81 in 2019.[11]

Does this mean the impact of Covid-19 has been exaggerated? In the grand march of progress, 2020 may later be seen as a blip. But that is not how events should be judged – they should be compared with contemporary expectations of what would have happened without the pandemic. And 2020 saw the biggest rise in age-standardized mortality rates for 70 years, since the major flu epidemic in 1951.

Numbers do not speak for themselves – appropriate context and comparison are essential for understanding whether they are 'big' or 'small'. Put in its proper context, 2020 was an historical outlier.

---

* These are standardized to the rates we would expect in a '2013 European Standard Population'.

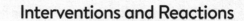

Interventions and Reactions

CHAPTER 16

What is the effect of measures against the spread of SARS-CoV-2?

Throughout the pandemic there has been continuing controversy about the effectiveness of measures taken against the virus, with some saying that 'lockdowns' have been unnecessary and harmful, and others arguing for more extreme measures that aim to eliminate the virus, claiming that they are linked to better health and economic outcomes.*[1]

Throughout this book we emphasize the importance of proper evaluation of interventions, focusing on controlled experiments using randomization; but restrictions have generally not been introduced according to a planned experimental design.† There was a small randomized trial of mask-wearing,[2] but it looked at protection of the wearer,[3] which is not the primary purpose of masks.‡ Operating-theatre

---

* The study referred to in note 1, comparing the outcomes of OECD countries that took an 'elimination' vs a 'mitigation' strategy, says: 'Although all indicators favour elimination, our analysis does not prove a causal connection between varying pandemic response strategies and the different outcome measures.' The title of the paper is not so cautious about attributing causation: 'SARS-CoV-2 elimination, not mitigation, creates best outcomes for health, the economy, and civil liberties'.

† An exception is the carefully designed UK programme for reopening large events, which had a strong scientific framework.

‡ Social media posts claiming this trial meant that 'masks do not work' were branded as misinformation by Facebook.

staff do not wear masks for self-protection; the only person without a mask is the patient.

Laboratory experiments have been valuable in assessing the impact of measures such as improved ventilation, physical distancing and face coverings on the spread of viral particles, but these studies cannot directly measure the impact of the spread through populations. So researchers have simply had to observe what countries did and measure the outcomes. These can seem obvious; just by examining the broad patterns of events in the UK, we can easily see that the lockdowns preceded a reduction in Covid-19 cases and deaths. But we cannot easily judge whether lighter responses would have sufficed and, since interventions tend to be introduced together, it is unclear how to disentangle the multiple effects of social distancing, home working, school closures and so on.

Can we use statistics to estimate the effect of different interventions?

Individual countries took different approaches to handling the pandemic, and so researchers treat those differences as a form of 'natural experiment' and try to work out the effects of various measures. The first step is to examine the policies adopted, and fortunately the Oxford COVID-19 Government Response Tracker (OxCGRT)[4] team have collected international data and dates on interventions. These can be summarized as a 'Stringency Index', on a scale from 0 to 100, displayed in Figure 16-1 for four selected countries.

New Zealand pursued an elimination strategy, with early, extremely stringent measures which were later relaxed, although the spikes in its graph show the government coming

New Zealand initiated strict early action, whilst other nations maintained stringent government responses

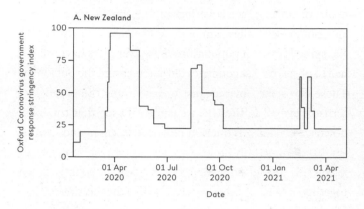

A. New Zealand

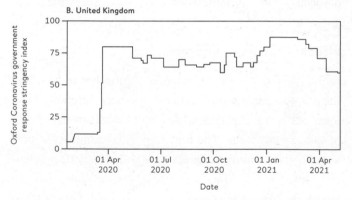

B. United Kingdom

Figure 16–1
Stringency Index for four different countries: a composite measure of nine indicators including school and workplace closures and travel bans, where 100 represents the strictest measures in some part of the country.

Source: Oxford Coronavirus Government Response Tracker project, via Our World in Data

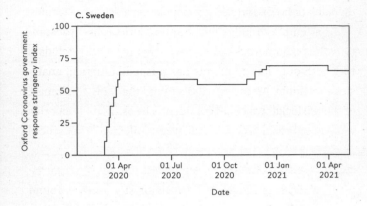

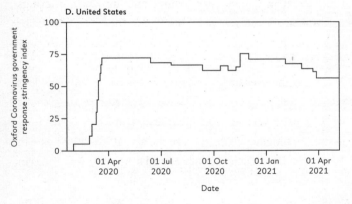

down hard on specific outbreaks. Sweden, although short of a full lockdown, kept a near-constant level of more modest restrictions. It is important to note that this index only deals with official policies, and so does not reflect voluntary actions by individuals or how rigorously the population abided by the rules.

In attempts to judge which interventions had substantial effects, numerous teams have tried to relate such data to health outcomes, but this has pushed statistical analysis to its limits. An early analysis found that only the impact of the full lockdown could confidently be estimated,[5] but this was strongly criticized.[6] A later study concluded that school closures and movement restrictions were effective in reducing transmission but was ambivalent about other measures,[7] while another major analysis of 41 countries found that school and university closures and limiting gatherings had the biggest effect,[8] and that 'when these interventions were already in place, issuing a stay-at-home order had only a small additional effect'.

These analyses are all related to the times when orders were issued, but people may have changed their behaviour in anticipation of explicit new rules; Figure 7–1 shows a fall in the UK's incidence rate before the actual lockdown date in January 2021,[9] coinciding with closed schools and changes in work and travel over the Christmas holidays.

Even with a mass of data, sometimes we just cannot find answers to our questions.

Could earlier lockdowns have saved lives?

Early mitigation in a pandemic can save lives. As a simplified example, imagine there are two countries, both with 100 initial cases. The reproduction number is 3, with on average a week between infections; one in 100 infected people later die. Suppose a lockdown reduces the reproduction number to 0.7, meaning infections decline with each 'generation' of the virus. If the first country locks down after the fourth generation, the total death toll from 15 generations of infections is 102. If the second country delays a week before lockdown, it is 305 – three times higher. Timing is critical.

Sophisticated models have come to similar conclusions,[10] estimating that locking down a week earlier, on 16 March 2020, would have reduced the first-wave death toll from around 37,000 to about 16,000 (8,900–26,800). Another week's delay would have increased deaths to over 100,000. Their model, however, only considers the two extreme alternatives of either simply giving advice to the public or a full lockdown.

What do the experts say?

Rather than relying on statistical analysis, an alternative approach is to bring experts together and combine informed judgements. The Scientific Advisory Group for Emergencies (SAGE) drew such conclusions in September 2020, summarized in Table 16–1.[11]

Table 16–1
Selected elements from the 'Summary of the effectiveness and harms of different non-pharmaceutical interventions' by SAGE in September 2020, listed in decreasing impact and 'confidence'. Their 'confidence' is a subjective assessment based on the quality of the underlying evidence and the agreement of the panel. Note that this reflects the understanding after the first wave alone and does not include other impacts, for example economic or social ones.

Intervention	Impact on transmission	Confidence
Stay at home order (lockdown), including school closure (with exceptions)	Very high	High
Short stay-at-home orders (Circuit-breakers)	Moderate	High
Closure of Higher Education	Moderate	High
Reducing household mixing indoors	Moderate	Medium
Closure of bars, pubs, cafes, and restaurants	Moderate	Medium
Mass school closure to prevent community transmission	Moderate	Low
Extend requirement for use of face covering indoors (e.g. shared offices, schools)	Low–moderate	
Impose local travel restrictions (e.g. 5-mile limit for non-essential travel)	Low–moderate	Low
Restrictions on outdoor gatherings, including prohibiting large events	Low	High
Prohibition of visitors to hospitals and care homes	Low	High
Restrict travel between UK nations or between subnational regions	Low	Moderate
Closure of non-essential retail	Low	Low–moderate
Increasing COVID security in workplaces and other settings	Low	Low
Requirement for use of face covering outdoors	Very low	High

SAGE ranked a full lockdown as the most effective measure. Unfortunately, it did not consider the additional effects of 'stay-at-home' orders, over and above everything else that could be done. Also notable is its lack of confidence in assessing the effect of school closures on transmission, and the low impact on transmission claimed for many of the interventions that we have been faced with. The high-confidence, 'very low' impact score given to wearing outdoor face coverings is reflected in this never having been a recommendation in the UK.

What is the effect of international travel and border controls?

Many countries have banned incomers from countries deemed to have high Covid-19 risks,[12] and this has had a huge impact on international travel and tourism. The number of visitors to the UK fell by 97% in April 2020,[13] compared to the same month in 2019.

The pandemic brought a massive change in foreign travel from the UK. Figure 16-2 first shows the very high levels of travel in normal times – between 5 and 11 million trips a month by UK residents, depending on the time of year – adding up to around 100 million trips a year. Then there was a precipitous plunge, falling by 96% in April–June 2020 compared to the second quarter of 2019.

Did all these travel restrictions have an impact on the spread of the virus? Back in February 2020, SAGE rejected travel restrictions,[14] saying that reducing imported infections by 50% would maybe delay the onset of any epidemic in the UK by about five days. In a similar vein, a prominent

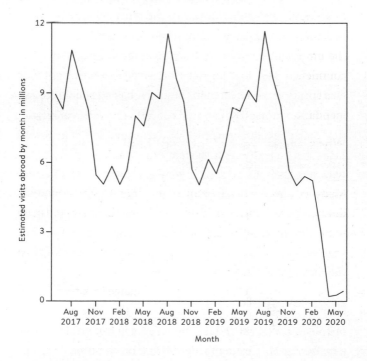

Estimated visits by UK residents abroad fell sharply in April 2020

Figure 16–2
UK residents' visits abroad by month, June 2017–June 2020.

Source: Office for National Statistics: Overseas travel and tourism, provisional: April to June 2020

team later concluded that stringent travel restrictions might have little impact,[15] 'except in countries with low COVID-19 incidence and large numbers of arrivals from other countries, or where epidemics are close to tipping points for exponential growth'. This does seem to have been the situation in the UK in March 2020 when, as we saw in Chapter 2, there was widespread introduction of the virus by European travellers.

Attitudes to travel restrictions subsequently changed, and an official study demonstrated the 'efficacy of travel restriction policy in reducing the onward transmission of imported cases'.[16] The traffic-light system of red–amber–green countries was then introduced in May 2021, when the situation was very different to that in 2020, since any deferment in introducing new infections allowed more of the population to be vaccinated. The delay in categorizing India as 'red' has therefore proved controversial, as it is likely to have sped up the introduction of the Delta (B.1.617.2) variant.

Does contact-tracing work?

People in contact with an infected person have a higher risk of infection. If contacts are infected, those people become another link in a chain of transmission. Contact-tracing is about breaking that chain by identifying people who have been in contact with an infected person.[17]

There are two main types of contact-tracing. *Backward* contact-tracing is when tracers seek to identify the source of infection, which requires considerable resources but has been successful in dealing with the spread of HIV. South Korean officials traced more than 5,000 Covid-19 cases back to meetings of a religious sect, whose leader was later arrested for hindering contact-tracing.[18]

The UK focused on *forward* contact-tracing, in which positive cases are interviewed and their recent contacts traced and told to isolate. Table 16–2 features key summaries of the weekly management information published by NHS Test and Trace in England.[19]

At the peak of the pandemic at the turn of 2020–21, nearly 390,000 people a week were transferred to the system. They identified around 740,000 close contacts, most of whom were asked to self-isolate.* In April 2021, the ONS asked people if they followed self-isolation requirements:[20] an estimated four in five (84%) claimed to do so, although to admit otherwise would have been to acknowledge breaking the law.

In England in early 2021, only about one in 10 contacts of a positive case later tested positive (the secondary attack rate).[21] So most contacts were likely to be uninfected, but all had to self-isolate, with no ability to escape the order through a negative test. Furthermore, the final row of Table 16–2 shows that the median time between a case showing symptoms and asking their contacts to isolate was more than four days, and rose to around six days in autumn 2020, which could give time for those contacts to spread the virus.

All of which raises the question: what has been the effect of telling millions of people to self-isolate, many more than once? The evidence is scanty. A probabilistic model sought

---

* Up to November 2020, tracers would have to contact each member of a household separately. After then, cases could inform others in their household of the need to isolate; tracers could mark those contacts as 'complete'. This methodological change led to a sudden jump in the proportion of close contacts reached from about 60% to over 90%.

Measure	Total (28 May 2020 to 5 May 2021)	Peak weekly value	Peak week (start date)
Number of people transferred to contact tracing system	3,862,252	388,150	31 December 2020
% people reached and asked to provide details of recent close contacts	87%	92%	18 March 2021
Number of people reached and asked to provide details of recent close contacts	3,345,441	341,685	31 December 2020
% who provided details for one or more close contacts	78%	85%	18 March 2021
Number of close contacts identified	8,264,952	737,044	31 December 2020
% close contacts reached and asked to self-isolate	82%	94%	21 January 2021[a]
Number of close contacts reached and asked to self-isolate	6,801,493	683,359	31 December 2020
Median time in hours from a case first observing symptoms to recent contacts being asked to self-isolate	102 (weighted average)	142	1 October 2020

a   NHS Test and Trace England report a peak percentage of 93.6% in three consecutive weeks, starting in the week commencing 21 January 2021.

Table 16–2
NHS Test and Trace England statistics for 28 May 2020–5 May 2021, with peak weeks. The total value for median delay between symptomatic cases and self-isolation orders is the authors' calculation, using a weighted average.

to estimate relative changes in the reproduction number due to testing-related interventions,[22] and estimated an 18%–33% reduction in R_t compared to only giving guidance for social distancing and imposing no self-isolation. Almost all the estimated benefit was from requiring those with a positive test to self-isolate, rather than any tracing of contacts.

There are digital enhancements to manual contact-tracing methods.[23] The NHS COVID-19 app had over 16 million regular users in late 2020, with the aim of notifying people if they had been near others with confirmed infections for at least 15 minutes. An average case 'pinged' four contacts, and overall only around 6% of people pinged went on to become cases. Both modelling and analytical approaches to assessing the NHS COVID-19 app suggest a benefit in England and Wales,[24] roughly averting one case per person sharing their contacts.

Assessing the effects of individual anti-transmission measures presents a challenging statistical problem. It is not answerable with confidence from available data, and there have only been meagre attempts at systematic evaluation. We can be confident that lockdowns have had an impact, but arguments will continue about whether less restrictive measures could be appropriate in a future pandemic.

What have been the collateral effects of the measures against Covid-19?

In early 2020, it would have been unthinkable to most of us that we would soon face a ban on most social contact with friends and family, the cessation of nearly all international travel, the shutting down of workspaces and schools, and so on. People have accepted and supported these measures, and radically altered their behaviour. These dramatic changes may have helped prevent the spread of the virus, but what have been the collateral harms, and possibly the benefits?

We will look at the impact on well-being and mental health and on the economy later, but first let's consider our non-Covid-19 health.

Have people been going to hospital?

Despite official encouragement to continue to seek medical care, normal health care suffered severe disruption. In Chapter 9 we saw how huge numbers of elective operations were cancelled, and there has also been a sharp reduction in other hospital referrals, possibly due to the reluctance of GPs to refer, anxiety and perceived risks of infection, as well as reduced hospital capacity through reorganization to cope with Covid-19 patients. For example, a study of English hospitals estimated that in March and April 2020 over 7,000 fewer people than the 2019 monthly average were admitted with suspected heart attack or unstable angina.[1]

The first part of the pandemic produced an unprecedented halving of visits to Accident and Emergency (A&E),[2] and even in May 2020 visits were a third below normal. Some changes could be considered positive: there was a sharp 65% drop in injuries, with an even greater fall in minor sporting or playground injuries.

There were reductions in elective cancer diagnoses in April and May 2020,[3] for breast (30% below normal), colon (39%), prostate (64%), and cervix (32%). Cancer investigations fell, with colonoscopies and gastroscopies at less than 10% of normal rates, and there were major falls in chemotherapy and radiotherapy. Even in the second wave, there was an 8% drop in the number of people starting cancer treatment in January 2021,[4] compared with the same month in 2020. Fortunately, there is no sign yet of excess cancer deaths (at the time of writing in May 2021), although this may only become apparent in subsequent years.[5]

What has happened to flu?

As we've already discussed in Chapter 3 and Chapter 15, the 'original' SARS-CoV-2 is far more infectious than seasonal influenza, with a basic reproduction number R_0 of around 3, compared to 1.3–1.5 for seasonal flu. If lockdowns and other measures are sufficient to bring R for SARS-CoV-2 down below one, then they should certainly be sufficient to crush flu.

That seems to have happened. Southern Hemisphere countries such as South Africa, Australia and Chile saw historically low levels of flu over their 2020 winter.[6] Figure 17–1

Flu remains suppressed, with Covid-19 admission rates in England rising until January 2021

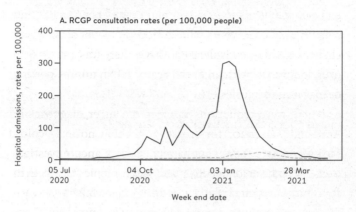

A. RCGP consultation rates (per 100,000 people)

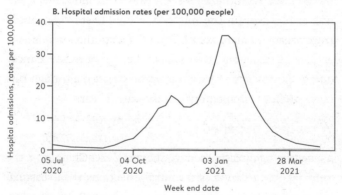

B. Hospital admission rates (per 100,000 people)

Figure 17–1

Consultation rates for influenza-like illnesses with GPs in England (graph A). Provisional hospital admission rates (graph B) are from SARI Watch.

A. —— Covid-19　　—— Influenza-like　　----- Influenza-like (2018–19)
B. —— Covid-19　　—— Influenza

Source: PHE Weekly national influenza and Covid-19 surveillance report, week 18 2021: National flu report data: 5 March 2020 (week 10)

reveals that in the winter of 2020–21, there were minimal consultations with GPs for influenza-like symptoms, and hospital admission rates with flu were near zero in England.[7]

Over recent years, seasonal flu is estimated to have killed between 4,000 (2018–19) and 22,000 (2017–18) people. The absence of flu in the winter of 2020–21 saved thousands of lives, and partially explains the below-average non-Covid-19 deaths seen throughout the second wave (Chapter 11).

Have there been fewer road casualties?

Figure 17–2 illustrates what happened when people travelled less; UK road casualties dropped sharply by around 70% in April 2020.[8] Japan showed a slightly different pattern: traffic reduced, and accidents went down, but deaths did not reduce by so much – people appeared to take advantage of empty roads to drive faster.[9] There is a suggestion that this occurred in the first half of 2020 in the UK, when the proportion of all casualties that were deaths reached a higher level (1.3%) than any in the previous 10 years.

Remember the 'bump' in mortality rates between the ages of 15 and 29 shown in Figure 12–2? That has been mitigated during the pandemic. In England and Wales in 2020, there were over 300 fewer death registrations for people in this age group compared with the average over the previous five years.* One putative explanation is reduced accidents and violence, and it means that due to the pandemic there are 300 fewer grieving families. These families do not know who

---

* Average deaths registered for 15–29-year-olds between 2015 and 2019: 2,692 men and 1,199 women. In 2020, 2,467 men and 1,114 women died.

Provisional estimates in Great Britain suggest a large fall in road casualties in April to June 2020

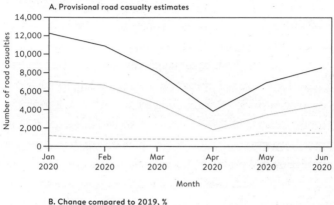

A. Provisional road casualty estimates

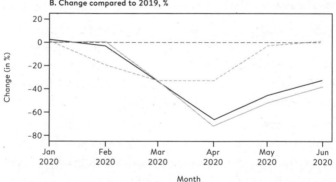

B. Change compared to 2019, %

Figure 17–2

The Department for Transport reports road casualties by different types of road user, covering both killed and injured, between January and June 2020. Graph A shows overall number of casualties, graph B shows the change from 2019.

Road user type

——— All road users   ——— Car users   - - - - Pedal cyclists

Source: Department for transport: Reported road casualties by road user type, first half 2020

they are, in contrast to the 115 families of those in this age group who died with Covid-19. The pandemic, and the measures taken against it, saved the lives of more young people than it killed.

Other impacts of reduced human activity are likely to be beneficial. Images showing that 'nature is healing' (including false claims about dolphins in Venetian canals)[10] spread online. Less transport meant reduced pollution,[11] with levels of nitrogen oxide (NOx) falling by around 40% during the second quarter of 2020 compared to the same months in 2019. Lower air pollution is also plausibly helping the bee population.[12] Worldwide, it's estimated that CO_2 emissions fell by 7% in 2020, but climate models suggest this will have had negligible effect on climate change.*[13]

What has been the effect of school closures?

In an article summarizing the potential harms to nearly 9 million children in the UK who have experienced school closures, researchers wrote: 'Children have least to gain and most to lose from school closures. This pandemic has seen an unprecedented intergenerational transfer of harm and costs from elderly socioeconomically privileged people to disadvantaged children.'[14] Despite the efforts of teachers and parents, there will have been substantial – but so far unquantified – harms to children in terms of their education, mental health and socialization.

Educational disruption can have long-term impacts.

---

* This is partly because reductions in air pollution tend to increase global temperature, since tiny particles can help reflect sunlight.

The shadow of the pandemic is cast far in the future, and there will be numerous attempts to estimate the impact of the pandemic through statistical analysis.

How has behaviour changed during the pandemic?

A pandemic has an enormous impact on what we do, whether in response to government rules and guidance, because of social awareness and peer pressure, personal feelings of fear or anxiety, or even just being sensible. The way we work, travel, educate our children, meet friends and family or relax have all changed. Less normal activities, such as crime and violence, have also been affected.

Here we look at the data on some of the extraordinary behavioural changes experienced since March 2020.

Have people adhered to the guidelines?

The first instructions in England to stay at home if you had Covid-19 symptoms were on 12 March 2020. Since then, rules and guidelines have come thick and fast, and people largely report having following them. In May 2021, responses to an ONS survey[1] indicated in the previous seven days:

- 88% had 'always' or 'often' washed their hands with soap and water after returning home from public places
- 97% used a face covering outside their home

- 79% maintained distance when meeting up with those outside of their support bubble, either 'always' or 'often'
- 83% avoided physical contact outside their home.*

Aside from face coverings (estimated to have been used by 28% in May 2020, when people were first advised to wear them), these percentages were high throughout the pandemic. Should we believe the numbers? There are reasons to be doubtful; high proportions may reflect **social desirability bias**, giving answers that would be viewed favourably by others. There is also **recall error**: people may not remember each instance of non-compliance.

There seems to have been a lot of curtain-twitching as people watched what their neighbours were up to. Over half (50%–54%) of respondents to the telephone-based Crime Survey for England and Wales had spotted others breaching restrictions,[2] although only a small proportion (3%–8%) of these said they reported those breaches to police, as most offences were considered trivial. But put together, this suggests that around one in 20 of the adult population had reported someone else to the police for breaching restrictions.

Overwhelming popular consent meant the rules did not require heavy policing: only 32,329 relevant Fixed Penalty Notices (FPNs) were issued in England and Wales between March and December 2020.[3] That including 196 FPNs for holding a gathering of more than 30 people, and 958 for not wearing a face covering. To put this in perspective, about

---

* When projected to the general population, the margins of error on these estimates are at most +/- 3%.

7,700 FPNs for motor vehicle offences are typically issued *every day* in England and Wales.[4]

How has work changed?

Even before the stay-at-home order of 23 March 2020, the Prime Minister's speech on 16 March included an instruction for 'people to start working from home where they possibly can'.[5] There are many workers who cannot work from home, and the proportion of working adults who did their job at least partly from home hovered around 60% during the peak of the lockdowns, falling to around 40% in the summer of 2020.

Meetings and social events shifted to online tools. Zoom meeting participants increased from 10 million in December 2019 to over 300 million in April 2020.[6] Microsoft Teams went from 20 million daily active users in 2019 to 115 million by the fourth quarter of 2020.[7] We could not find statistics on how often people were asked to unmute themselves.

Where have people been going?

People were told to travel only if necessary. Rather than directly asking them what they were doing, automatic data was collected from mobile-phone users. Using location data provided by Android phone users who turned on their location history (who may not be representative), Google created a mobility index, shown in Figure 18–1.

Relative to early 2020,[9] travel to workplaces more than halved, as people spent more time at home. Parks were, predictably, more popular during the summer. As we saw in

Since the start of the pandemic, visitors to work-places remained under baseline values

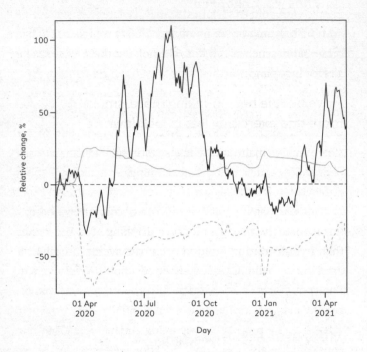

Figure 18–1

Changes in Google mobility data between February 2020 and May 2021 (rolling seven-day average). Each weekday has a different baseline value, which is the median value in the five-week period from 3 January to 6 February.[8] The residential category measured time spent at home, rather than changes in visitors.

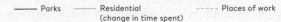

——— Parks   ——— Residential   ----- Places of work
                 (change in time spent)

Source: Google Covid-19 Community mobility trends, via Our World in Data

Chapter 17, reduction in travel led to falls in road casualties – a collateral benefit of the lockdown.

People were told to socially distance, isolate with symptoms and work from home if possible. Nobody told us to change other habits, such as drinking alcohol, but these may also be altered by a pandemic.[10]

Have people been drinking more, smoking more and exercising less in lockdown?

There are two main ways of investigating drinking habits: ask people how much they are consuming, or measure alcohol purchases.

The Alcovision survey of over 80,000 drinkers found,[11] unsurprisingly, that people were drinking at home rather than in pubs during lockdown, but the average number of drinking days did not change. The Alcohol Consumption in England project estimated that the proportion of people reporting high-risk drinking rose substantially during the first wave, but the proportion reporting cutting down on their consumption also went up.[12] Lockdown effects, like the effects of the virus, vary hugely. But although there have been changes in patterns of drinking, when we look at paid duty, the provisional total amount of alcohol consumed appeared to remain stable.[13]

Smoking dropped in 2020 compared to 2019, although this was in line with the existing trend.[14] In the Smoking Toolkit Study, more reported they were attempting to quit, rising from around 30% pre-lockdown to nearly 40% by September 2020.

When it comes to getting off the sofa and exercising, the Active Lives survey found lockdowns favoured the sofa.[15] During the first wave, around 3 million fewer adults were 'active' (doing at least two and a half hours a week of 'moderate-intensity' exercise), while the 'inactive' number (less than 30 minutes a week) rose by a similar amount.

With restrictions limiting leisure, and greater numbers working at home, exercising outside became more common. In May 2020, 36% of Natural England's People and Nature survey said they were spending more time outside, and by July 2020 that share rose to 46%.[16]

Have people turned to illegal drugs?

The European Monitoring Centre for Drugs and Drug Addiction (EMCDDA) has the interesting task of following activity on three popular dark-net drug markets.[17] It reported an overall increase in activity related to cannabis use since the beginning of 2020, although there was a decline in demand for party drugs, presumably because of the lack of parties. There was also a decrease in dealers buying high volumes due to resale difficulties, and a corresponding increase in smaller volumes for personal use.

Have people turned to crime?

We must be careful when using police reports of crime. These are notorious for fluctuations depending on how reporting is being done at the time, and indeed were de-designated as 'official statistics' in 2014. With these warnings, the ONS reported a sharp drop in police-recorded crimes in April–June 2020,[18] from the 2019 level of about 510,000 a month down to around 420,000 (a 19% decrease). However, by September police-recorded crimes were only 4% below their 2019 level.

Figure 18–2 shows the changes in different types of recorded crime in April 2020 compared to 2019 levels. There was a steep drop in sexual offences, robbery (with a threat or actual violence) and theft. Other types of crime fell to a lesser extent, except drug offences which were up 50%. That increase probably reflects heightened police activity rather than greater criminal activity - there was a marked increase in stop and search by the Metropolitan Police during the first lockdown,[19] primarily because of suspected drugs misuse, nearly doubling to over 40,000 in May 2020.

What about domestic violence?

Figure 18–2 shows that, by April 2020, violent offences fell by about 10% compared to April 2019. But against this trend, the ONS reported that between March and June 2020 there was a 9% increase in domestic abuse-related offences, compared to the same months a year earlier.[20] Such offences have unfortunately seen a steady rise in recent years, so that increase may not be wholly due to the pandemic.

Many victim services have reported increased demand, particularly after restrictions eased and victims presumably felt they could safely seek help after being constrained within their homes. Refuge, the charity which runs the National Domestic Abuse Helpline, reported a 61% increase in calls and contacts between April 2020 and February 2021, compared with the first three months of 2020,[21] while there was a sevenfold increase in visits to their website following

In April 2020, almost all categories of police-recorded crimes decreased compared to 2019

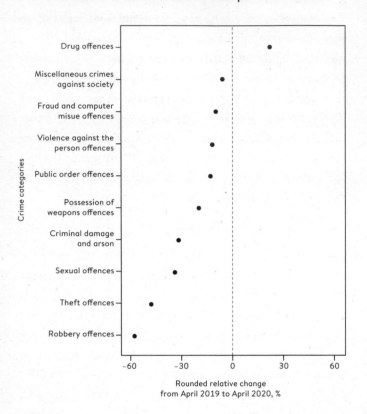

Figure 18–2

The numbers of crimes in each category recorded by police in England and Wales at the height of lockdown in April 2020 as a proportion of those in April 2019. These figures exclude Greater Manchester Police.

● The increase in drug offences reflects increased policing activity in hotspots

Source: Office for National Statistics: Crime in England and Wales: year ending September 2020

the #YouAreNotAlone awareness campaign launched in April 2020.[22]

Restriction to our homes was inevitably accompanied by many alterations in behaviour. Much was in line with expectations, whether a decrease in physical activity or an increase in domestic violence, while Pornhub reported an increase in traffic during the enforced inactivity of the pandemic.[23] Some changes, such as greater home working, may be permanent, while others may revert to their normal trends. It is too soon to say.

What has happened to mental health and well-being?

Wars leave scars on a nation: graves, shattered families and broken buildings. Pandemics also cast a grim shadow. Alongside the suffering and death there is disrupted schooling, enforced inactivity, people are cut off from loved ones and businesses stunted. It would be remarkable if mental health and well-being did not suffer.

The ONS Opinions and Lifestyle (OPN) Survey is a weekly survey of over 4,000 adults in Great Britain.[*1] There are four main questions about well-being – satisfaction with life, happiness, life being worthwhile, and anxiety – which are asked using the phrases shown in Figure 19–1, on a scale from 0 ('not at all') to 10 ('completely').[2] Where would you put yourself today?

The baseline figures suggest the British are usually fairly satisfied with life, with well-being ratings above the average for the EU.[3] But life satisfaction declined from the start of the pandemic, reaching a low in January 2021. Estimated

---

* Samples are drawn from people who have answered previous national surveys run by the ONS; the survey is mainly carried out online, with an option for telephone interviews. All these figures are estimates with margins of sampling error, around +/- 0.1 % around the central number.

Estimated life satisfaction in Great British adults has yet to recover to its pre-lockdown level

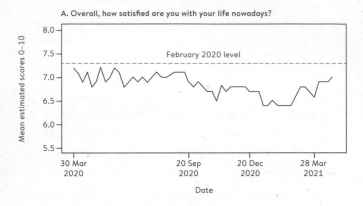

A. Overall, how satisfied are you with your life nowadays?

February 2020 level

B. Overall, how happy did you feel yesterday?

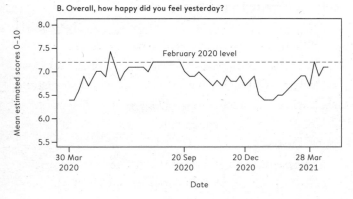

February 2020 level

Figure 19–1

Trends in the estimated mean scores (0–10) for the four well-being questions in the ONS Opinions and Lifestyle Survey for adults between March 2020 and March 2021: life satisfaction, happiness, life being worthwhile and anxiety.

Source: Office for National Statistics – Opinions and lifestyle surveys

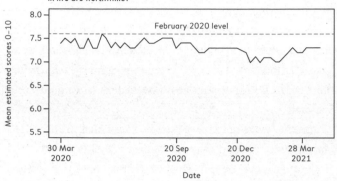

C. Overall, to what extent do you feel that the things you do in life are worthwhile?

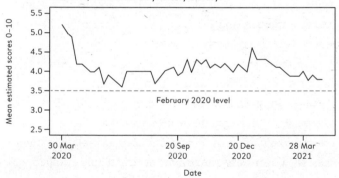

D. Overall, how anxious did you feel yesterday?

average happiness was blunted, recovering in the summer, then hitting a nadir in January 2021. The average feeling that things in life are worthwhile oscillated under its February 2020 level, before dropping in January 2021. Reported anxiety attained its zenith in March 2020, when the estimated average score was 5.2. By the end of June 2020, anxiety had dropped down to an average 3.6, close to its February 2020 level. Anxiousness bubbled up again in January 2021, when there were national stay-at-home orders in England and Scotland.

Another wave of the OPN survey found that in July 2019–March 2020, around one in 10 adults (8%–12%) reported moderate to severe depressive symptoms,* but by June 2020 that proportion had nearly doubled to 19% (16%–22%).[4] Adults aged under 40, women, people unable to afford unexpected expenses and disabled people were more likely to report depressive-like symptoms.

The OPN survey also showed that the proportion of adults reporting they were 'often' or 'always' lonely was about 5% in April–May 2020,[5] and by winter that increased to around 7%, higher in dense urban areas. Of those who said the pandemic affected their well-being, 39% blamed loneliness, with over three times more young people citing loneliness than older people.

Increased anxiety fed through to calls to mental health charities. As ITV reported in May 2020: 'The number of calls

---

* Respondents say whether each of eight problems bothered them in the past two weeks 'not at all' (scored 0) to 'nearly every day' (scored 3). The total score is out of 24: with 10 or more meaning the person has 'moderate to severe symptoms'.

to the charity SANE's telephone helpline has increased by 200% since the lockdown began."[6] Unfortunately that headline was misinterpreted, with some social media accounts asserting that the number of people taking their own lives had increased by that much.[7]

The ONS publishes provisional statistics on registered suicides every three months,[8] and death registrations where people have taken their own lives were similar in July–September 2020 compared to previous years, and lower in April to June. However, it's important to remember that there are often considerable delays if there is an inquest into how a death happened, and the pandemic affected coroner services.

To overcome delays, researchers established a real-time surveillance system of suspected suicides in several parts of England covering about 13 million people.[9] Following the lockdown, the monthly average number of suspected suicides fell. There were 125.7 per month in January–March 2020, which went down to 121.3 per month in April–October 2020. A similar pattern of little to no change was seen in other high-income countries.[10] In wartime, anxiety rises but suicides do not increase, and may even go down. It is plausible that the same happened in the pandemic.

This has been an incredibly difficult time for many, and some may find it challenging to re-enter society as it returns to some form of normality. There will be an invisible pool of continued ill-health.

What have been people's attitudes and beliefs about the pandemic?

We've looked at statistics about how our behaviour, physical and mental health have been affected by the pandemic. Rather more difficult to measure, but vitally important, is the impact on our feelings, whether about the virus and the interventions taken against it, or about whom we have trusted, or what claims we have believed. Once again, this illustrates the huge variety – both physical and mental – of responses to a novel situation.

How do people vary in the way they perceive the risk from Covid-19?

In the UK, the pandemic came, withered in the summer of 2020, and then returned with a vengeance. A study revealed that public perception of Covid-19 risks followed a similar pattern: falling after the first wave, and then rising as the second wave took hold.[1] The researchers found that the five strongest predictors of perceiving higher risk from Covid-19 were:

- a 'communitarian world view': belief in the importance of society, rather than individualism

- 'personal efficacy': what you do makes a difference
- 'pro-sociality': doing things for the good of society
- trusting in science
- being female

with, of course, their opposites linked to perceiving lower risk from Covid-19. All these variables were more important than personal experience or political affiliation, and may impact on people's relationships with family, friends and acquaintances, and their varying attitudes about whether there has been too much or too little fuss made about the virus.

How do people feel about lockdown and mask-wearing?

There has been extraordinarily widespread support for the anti-virus measures. In April 2021, the ONS estimated that 83% (81%–85%) strongly supported or tended to support lockdown measures where they lived.[2] Only 2% strongly opposed. An Ipsos MORI poll in January 2021 found that nearly half believed the measures were not strict enough – and only 9% thought they were too strict.[3]

The Ipsos MORI survey found that, if confirmed cases rose, about three-quarters (76%) strongly supported or tended to support compulsory mask-wearing at work. Around 61% felt mask-wearing should always be mandatory outdoors, despite little evidence that it would slow transmission. There was notable support for even stronger restrictions if the pandemic got worse: about 34% endorsed the idea that people should only be allowed out with an official pass.

Who is trusted?

Scientists played a prominent role throughout the pandemic. Trust in scientists has always been high in the UK, just below that for doctors and nurses, and this trust held up well in 2020 with 60% of respondents considering scientists trustworthy, and only 12% untrustworthy.[4] These figures were slightly less favourable for scientists advising the government, at 55% versus 15% respectively.

In contrast, trust in the UK government fell from 65% of respondents being 'very or somewhat confident' in their handling of a pandemic in February 2020 down to 37% in January 2021.[5] There may be some restoration in confidence as restrictions unwind and vaccines roll.

Do people believe misinformation about Covid-19?

There is a lot of dubious information online, much going beyond reasonable scepticism into misinformation. An analysis back in March 2020 found that of the top Covid-19-related videos on YouTube, over a quarter contained misleading information and those had over 62 million views worldwide.[6] This could be important: a randomized experiment found that exposure to misinformation about vaccines led to an estimated six-point reduction in intention to get vaccinated.[7] The WHO runs a 'Mythbusters' page containing counter-arguments to Covid-19 misinformation, ranging from the dangers of injecting bleach to the lack of benefit of eating garlic to ward off the virus.[8]

In this book we have tried to deal with some misleading

Claim	% rating the claim more reliable than not
The coronavirus was bioengineered in a military lab in Wuhan.	25%
Being able to hold your breath for 10 seconds or more without coughing or discomfort is a good self-check test for whether you have the coronavirus	17%
The coronavirus is part of a global effort to enforce mandatory vaccination.	15%
Gargling salt water or lemon juice reduces the risk of infection from Coronavirus	11%
The new 5G network may be making us more susceptible to the virus	9%
Breathing in hot air through your mouth and nose (e.g. from a hair dryer) kills the coronavirus as it can only live in cool places.	7%

Table 20–1
Proportion of 2,200 UK respondents rating each claim as more reliable than not (rating 5,6 or 7 on a scale running from '1: very unreliable' to '7: very reliable').

claims, but how much support have these had? A multi-country online survey (conducted by DS's colleagues)* asked people how reliable they considered the six claims in Table 20–1, which shows the proportion in the UK thinking each claim was more reliable than not.[9]

The suggestion that the virus was bioengineered in Wuhan was thought more reliable than not by a quarter of respondents.† The idea that 5G networks made us more susceptible to the virus was supported by about 9%; these figures were higher in Spain and Mexico.

The researchers found that those who believed these claims tended to self-report less compliance with Covid-19 guidance, and increased hesitancy about then-hypothetical vaccines. The most important factors linked to 'resilience' to such claims were higher trust in scientists and, interestingly, higher numeracy skills.

We cannot confidently conclude that the observed link between numeracy and resilience to misinformation is causal. But it encourages the idea that greater 'data literacy' could bring critical awareness of the dubious claims in circulation.

---

* The countries were the UK, Ireland, the US, Spain and Mexico.

† Since this survey was conducted, the possibility of a leak from a scientific research laboratory has been discussed more seriously, but this is distinct from the idea of a military-engineered bio-weapon.

CHAPTER 21

What has been the effect on the economy?

The year since the start of the pandemic was like no other. Governments enforced rules limiting physical contact, people worked from home, pubs and shops closed and jobs were lost, and, rather than going out and spending money, people sat at home and watched Netflix. All these changes had dramatic effects on economic measures.

How did the pandemic affect employment?

In his address on 16 March 2020, the Prime Minister told everyone to avoid 'pubs, clubs, theatres and other social venues'.[1] This was detrimental if you worked in those sectors, while the stay-at-home order a week later resulted in most shops closing. New rules meant that some jobs could not continue, but British companies could claim wages from the UK government through the 'furlough' scheme.[2] From a statistical perspective, that meant people technically remained employed under the International Labour Organization definition.

Figure 21–1 shows the pandemic reversing recent positive trends in different employment metrics, returning to the levels of around 2017. Future trends, particularly after the end of the furlough scheme, are very uncertain.

There was an estimated quarterly decrease in the unemployment rate, while the economic inactivity rate increased

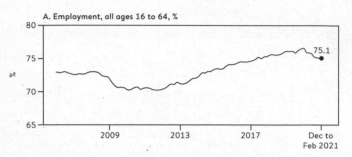

A. Employment, all ages 16 to 64, %

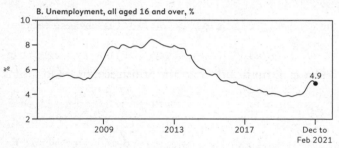

B. Unemployment, all aged 16 and over, %

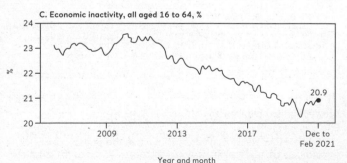

C. Economic inactivity, all aged 16 to 64, %

Year and month

The estimated redundancy rate shot up, from about four in 1,000 employees in the quarter before the pandemic to over 12 in 1,000 in the final quarter of 2020. That was higher than in the 2008–09 financial crisis.

Even if counted as employed, furloughed people were not at work and so there were drastic impacts on total hours worked, as recorded in the Labour Force Survey.[3] Figure 21–2 shows that in early 2020, all employed people in the UK worked an estimated total of 1,050 million hours each week, but by April–June 2020 that fell to about 840 million hours each week. At the end of 2020, the number of hours worked had only partially recovered.

How was gross domestic product affected?

A nation's gross domestic product (GDP) is a key economic indicator. By April–June 2020, the British economy had shrunk by over one-fifth, compared to its level in the fourth quarter of 2019.[4] But this pain was not uniform across industries.

The UK has a services-led economy, and Figure 21–3 shows how these were variously affected by the pandemic. Accommodation and food services were the hardest hit in the second quarter, shrinking to 15% of the 2019 Q4 level.

[Facing page] Figure 21–1
'Unemployment' counts people who were actively seeking work in the last four weeks and can start work in the next two weeks. 'Economically inactive' means people who are neither employed nor unemployed. The unemployment rate is the proportion of economically active people who are unemployed. All clear?

Source: Office for National Statistics: Labour Force Survey

The recovery in total actual weekly hours was impacted by new restrictions

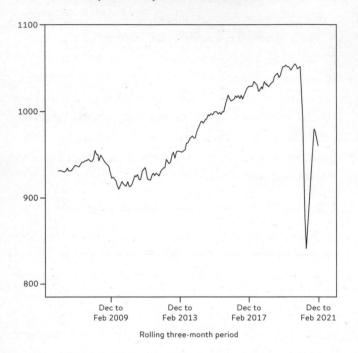

Rolling three-month period

Figure 21–2
UK estimated total actual weekly hours worked (all people aged 16 and over). In millions, seasonally adjusted.

Source: Office for National Statistics: Labour force survey

Services grew by a revised 17% in Q3 2020, but remained 9% under the Q4 2019 level

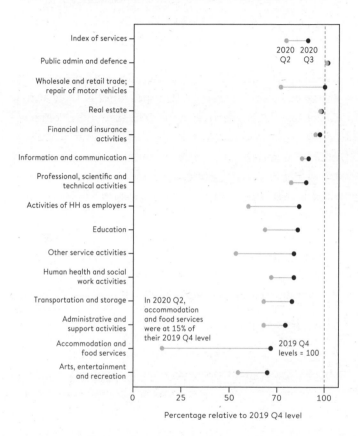

Figure 21–3

UK services gross domestic product index Q3 2020 (April–June) and Q4 2020 (July–September) compared to Q4 2019 (vertical dashed line).

Source: Office for National Statistics, GDP quarterly national accounts, July to September 2020

By the third quarter of 2020, there had been some recovery. Quarterly GDP growth was an estimated 16%. That is the largest single quarter of growth since quarterly records began in 1955. Despite the intrepid bounceback, the economy was still smaller than in the last quarter of 2019.

The UK reported the second-largest impact from the pandemic among the G7 countries, second only to Spain. However, national statistics institutes differ in the way they calculate GDP;[5] in particular, the ONS uses more volume of activity indicators (such as the number of operations in hospitals, which were hit hard by the pandemic) than others do. Using 'nominal' GDP, expressed in terms of value of activity, the UK's reduction is broadly comparable to those of other G7 countries.[6]

Due to fewer receipts and more claimants, government spending grew. In March 2021, UK public-sector net debt (excluding public-sector banks) stood at 98% of the nation's GDP, compared to 63% in 2010 and 31% in 2000.[7]

How did the pandemic change our spending?

The Covid-19 pandemic has accelerated trends in how we shop. The ONS reported a large fall in retail sales in March and April 2020, coinciding with the national stay-at-home order.[8] Rather predictably, digital retail sales grew, as shown in Figure 21–4.[9] Prior to 2020, it took seven years for the proportion of online sales to grow by 10 percentage points, and then in one year the digital share increased by 16 points. Amazon made US$8 billion profit in the first three months of 2021, more than double the previous year.[10]

This major acceleration in digital migration included a

Excluding auto fuels, the internet share of all sales reached a record proportion of 36% in February 2021

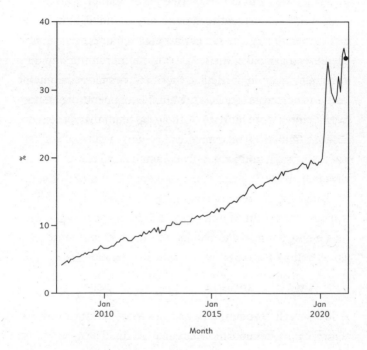

Figure 21–4
Estimated Internet share of sales value (all retail excluding auto fuel, seasonally adjusted) in Great Britain (%), for January 2008 to March 2021.

Source: Office for National Statistics: Monthly business survey - Retail sales inquiry, April 2021

rapid rise for stores which mostly sell food,[11] most likely due to concerns about visiting supermarkets, for which the digital share increased from 5% in January 2020 to 12% a year later.

Another component of this shift was in entertainment. With cinemas and other places closed, people turned to streaming services and computer games. Major films went directly on to these services without a cinema release. According to a Netflix letter to shareholders, the company acquired a net 36.6 million subscribers, representing an increase of 22% over its 2019 Q4 base.[12] Despite only launching in November 2019, Disney+ had amassed almost 95 million paid subscribers by 2 January 2021.[13] In the 2020–21 financial year, Nintendo sold 28.8 million Switch consoles, 37% more than the previous year.[14] This all meant a lot more time on the sofa.

As we climb out of the pandemic, economies should continue to improve. It is too soon to see the big picture, but there are likely to be permanent changes in how we work and shop. Young people, who have sacrificed so much while being at low risk themselves, face an even more uncertain future than they did before this virus came along.

Vaccines

How effective are the vaccines?

Vaccines work by training the body's own immune system to fight off the virus if it encounters it later; this training takes at least seven and sometimes 14 days. Right from the start of the pandemic, there had been hope of vaccines coming to rescue us from new waves. In an astonishing story of massively funded international scientific innovation, many vaccines were developed, tested and administered, and formed new topics of conversation – 'Which one did you get?'.[1]

The discussion of vaccines has been awash with numbers, with intense interest in how effective they are, how safe they are, who should get them first and what the gap should be between doses. Different countries have taken distinct approaches to procurement and roll-out. The UK Vaccine Task Force negotiated a beneficial contract with AstraZeneca to manufacture the vaccine first produced in Oxford, as well as ordering large numbers of other vaccines. All this had to be done before it was clear which vaccine candidates would be effective – a common practice being to 'de-risk' the pharmaceutical industry in order to massively accelerate development.

Late in 2020, the first reports started appearing with the trial findings of different vaccines against Covid-19, such as 'Moderna: Covid vaccine shows nearly 95% protection'.[2] What does that mean?

What is the 'efficacy' of the vaccines in clinical trials?

The crucial step for regulating new interventions are 'Phase III' clinical studies.[3] Volunteers are randomly allocated to receive either the vaccine or a control injection (a saline placebo or a different vaccine). Researchers follow the volunteers and check how many develop the disease and other important outcomes. We saw in Chapter 10 how such randomized controlled trials are the gold standard for assessing treatments, but vaccine trials have some special characteristics since, even in large trials, severe events like hospitalization are too rare to precisely estimate protection.[4] This means that trials measure, for example, the ability of the vaccine to reduce symptomatic disease at least seven days after the second dose, whereas this is not really the main outcome of practical interest.

Neither health-care staff nor the volunteers should know whether the jab is active or the control – volunteers may change their behaviours if they know which they got. Due to random assignment, researchers can then claim that observed differences – beyond those explicable by twists of chance – are due to the vaccine.

Vaccine efficacy is the relative change in having a disease in the vaccinated group,[5] compared against people without the vaccination in the same trial. Table 22–1 shows the calculation from the first Pfizer-BioNTech clinical trial.[6]

There are 170 Covid-19 cases: eight (0.043% of 18,198) are

	Pfizer-BioNTech	Placebo injection	Efficacy (95% uncertainty interval)
Number in each group	18,198	18,325	
Number of cases of Covid-19 at least 7 days after 2nd dose	8·	162	
Proportion getting the disease	0.043%	0.884%	95% (90% to 98%)

Table 22–1
Main results from randomized controlled trial of Pfizer-BioNTech vaccine; vaccine efficacy is estimated by 1 – 0.043/0.884 = 0.95.

in the vaccine group, and 162 (0.884% of 18,325) in the placebo group. The relative reduction from 0.884% to 0.043% is the claimed 95%. That is the central estimate of vaccine efficacy, with a **credible interval** of 90% to 98%, the width of which is determined by the (rather small) number of cases rather than the number of participants.

High efficacy becomes plain in the 'cumulative incidence' graph of new cases shown in Figure 22–1. The two groups have a similar rise in cases in the opening days, and then after around 10 days there are only a few further cases among vaccinated volunteers, while non-vaccinated cases continue to climb. As Randall Monroe (xkcd) said: 'Always try to get data that's good enough you don't need to do statistics on it.'[7]

Headline trial results for symptomatic disease are shown in Table 22–2 – other vaccine candidates, for example from Sanofi, have not yet reached Phase III trials. There are common claims that the vaccine trials demonstrated '100% efficacy' against severe outcomes, such as hospitalization.[16] That means no events occurred in the vaccinated group, but it is not a reliable estimate: in the Moderna trial, there were no Covid-19 deaths in the vaccinated group, but this was versus only one in the control group.

Table 22–2 should not be used to make simplistic comparisons, as these trials were carried out at different times, with different populations, designs and outcome measures. The vaccines also have different costs, storage demands and safety profiles, as we shall see in Chapter 23.

Covid-19 cases keep rising in the placebo group soon after the first dose

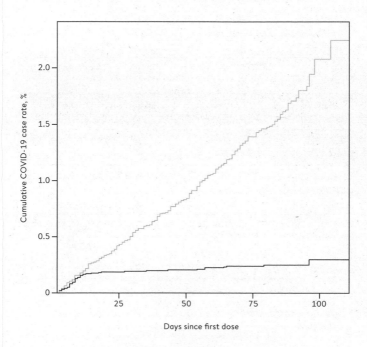

Figure 22–1

The cumulative incidence (%) of Covid-19 cases, from the day of the first dose in the Pfizer–BioNTech phase III trial, showing the deviation between the vaccinated and placebo groups after 10 days.

——— Vaccine   ——— Placebo

Graphical reconstruction.
Source: Pfizer/BioNTech/NEJM and FDA

Vaccine	Type*	Population	Estimated efficacy	95% interval
Pfizer–BioNTech[8] BNT162b2	mRNA	Mainly US	95%	90% to 98%
Oxford–AstraZeneca[9] ChAdOx1	Viral vector	US	76%	68% to 82%
Moderna[10] mRNA-1273	mRNA	US	94%	89% to 97%
Sputnik V[11] Gam-COVID-Vac	Viral vector	Russia	92%	86% to 95%
Novavax[12] NVX-CoV2373	Protein	UK	90%	80% to 95%
Johnson & Johnson[13] JNJ-78436735	Viral vector (single-dose)	US, South Africa, Latin America	66%	60% to 72%
Sinovac[14] Coronavac	Inactivated virus	Brazil and Turkey	51%	36% to 62%

* mRNA means 'messenger RNA'. Once these instructions are inside cells, cells use them to make the protein piece. The cells then display that piece on their surface and the body recognises it as foreign, which stimulates an immune response. Cells break down the mRNA after using its instructions. Viral vector vaccines use an edited version of a different and harmless virus. Those vectors enter a cell, causing it to produce the spike protein. In turn, our body recognises that the spike protein should not be there and develops antibodies to fight it. Protein subunit vaccines include harmless pieces of the virus to induce an immune response. Inactivated virus vaccine use viruses with destroyed genetic material (through heat, chemicals or radiation). These inactivated viruses cannot replicate, but still trigger an immune response.

Table 22–2
Summary of estimates of efficacy against symptomatic disease from clinical trials, in order of release.[15] Efficacy applies to variants circulating at the time of each trial, mainly 'wild-type'.

How effective are the vaccines in normal use?

Despite their confusing similarity, vaccine *effectiveness* is a different concept to *efficacy*. Researchers estimate efficacy in tightly controlled trials, which can exclude people like children, pregnant women, or those with compromised immune systems.[17] In contrast, **vaccine effectiveness** is about routine performance in the real world, where storage and administration may also matter.

In Chapter 10, we saw that 'real-world' data could suggest that a Covid-19 treatment was beneficial, but then be contradicted when tested in clinical trials. The order is different for vaccines: trials come first, and only after roll-out programmes start can we estimate how much vaccines reduce severe outcomes in practice.

But, as with observational data for treatments, we cannot just compare people who got a vaccine versus those who did not. These groups differ: roll-outs may prioritize older and more vulnerable people, and hesitant people may be at higher risk. People who are ill may not get the vaccine. So effectiveness studies adopt a range of designs and techniques to attempt fair comparisons.

An early **prospective cohort study**[18] followed the entire adult population of Scotland,[19] checking when people had a hospital admission with Covid-19. The analysis compared 1.3 million people with at least one dose of a vaccine to 3.1 million non-vaccinated people. The analysis tried to take possible **confounding** factors into account, including age, sex, deprivation and other medical conditions.

Figure 22–2 reveals that the effectiveness for preventing hospitalization with Covid-19 peaked four weeks after the first dose, at 91% (uncertainty interval 85%–94%) for Pfizer-BioNTech and 88% (75%–94%) for Oxford-AstraZeneca. It might look like the Pfizer vaccine was better, but the intervals show that would be unjustified. For the Oxford-AstraZeneca vaccine, effectiveness for over-80s was 81% (60%–91%). President Macron's claim about quasi-ineffectiveness (*quasi inefficace*) in older people was shown to be wrong.

Other designs include a **matched-control study** in Israel,[20] in which each person who had received the Pfizer-BioNTech vaccination was 'twinned' with a non-vaccinated control of the same age, sex, geography and other factors; their effectiveness estimates were similar to those above.

Reducing hospital admissions is important, but vaccines need also to protect against infection and transmission. A study of over 370,000 participants in the ONS Covid-19 Infection Survey showed that infections were reduced by 65% (60%–70%) after a single vaccination,[21] with one dose affording similar protection to a prior infection. The two vaccines (Pfizer-BioNTech and Oxford-AstraZeneca) had comparable effects. Protection against severe infection was even greater, as defined by lower cycle threshold values and symptoms.

Vaccination can reduce transmission in two ways. First, by preventing people from getting infected in the first place. Second, if vaccinated people tend to develop a weaker form of infection, then they might be less likely to transmit the virus. A study by Public Health England of over 500,000 households showed that the chance of an infected person

Scottish data suggests one dose of Covid-19 vaccines offer protection against admission

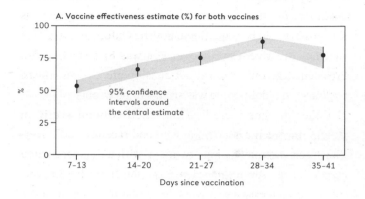

A. Vaccine effectiveness estimate (%) for both vaccines

95% confidence intervals around the central estimate

Days since vaccination

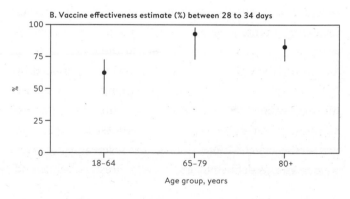

B. Vaccine effectiveness estimate (%) between 28 to 34 days

Age group, years

Figure 22–2

Vaccine effectiveness (for Pfizer–BioNTech and Oxford–AstraZeneca combined) for reducing hospitalization for different periods after a single vaccination, and for different age groups.

Source: Interim findings from first-dose mass Covid-19 vaccination roll-out and Covid-19 hospital admissions in Scotland: a national prospective cohort study (Lancet, 2021)

passing the virus to someone else in their household was reduced by nearly half if that infected person was vaccinated.[22]

These were encouraging results, particularly given the then dominance of the Alpha (B.1.1.7) variant in England. Even though these are observational studies, without the same reliability as clinical trials, they do indicate that vaccines reduce both viral transmission and severity, lowering cases and deaths.

What about new variants?

At the time of writing (May 2021), there was considerable uncertainty about the effectiveness of the vaccines against new variants. Preliminary work by Public Health England used a 'test-negative control' study* to estimate that the effectiveness of one dose in protecting against symptomatic disease fell from around 50% against the Alpha (B.1.1.7) variant to 33% against the Delta variant (B.1.617.2), while the effectiveness of two doses only experienced a small fall from 88% to 81%.[23] This suggests that a single dose has less than half the effectiveness of two doses against the Delta (B.1.617.2) variant and led to higher-risk groups having the gap between their vaccinations shortened from 12 weeks to eight weeks (see Chapter 25).

What has been the impact of the vaccines?

Public Health England regularly estimates total lives saved by the vaccination programme, modelling how many deaths

---

* This matches each person who tests positive with someone who tested negative at the same time, and then compares their vaccination histories; the idea is that this should control for all the factors that led them to seek a test.

from Covid-19 we would have expected without vaccines.[24] Up to 13 May 2021, assuming the vaccines were 81% effective at preventing death, they estimated that 13,200 deaths in over-60s had been averted, not including the indirect benefits from reduced infection and transmission. Other analyses compared trajectories of different age groups and showed death rates in older groups dropping faster than for younger people awaiting vaccination.[25]

As we learn to live with this virus, the vaccines may need to be adjusted for new variants, just as happens to flu vaccines, and they will not have to go through the regulatory process each time. The development and roll-out of the Covid-19 vaccines has been an extraordinary success story – it is chilling to imagine our situation without them.

How safe are the vaccines?

Some anxiety about new vaccines is understandable – they have been developed fast, and given in vast numbers to healthy people, not all of whom may benefit. There has been intense interest in announcements from regulatory bodies monitoring adverse reactions. Different countries came to a variety of decisions, based on varying interpretations of the data and attitudes to risk.

When millions of people are vaccinated, many apparent **adverse events** will happen within a few weeks by chance. People will have heart attacks, strokes or get run over by buses. The problem lies in discerning genuine side effects from events that may have happened anyway – call it luck, chance or fate, it is difficult to incorporate into our thinking.

Anxiety about vaccines was raised by a much-publicized paper in 1999 falsely asserting a causal link between the MMR vaccine and autism. But these claims were based on an un-controlled series of 12 children, with speculative conclusions from fraudulent results,[1] and later analyses showed that the incidence of autism after vaccination was indistinguishable from the rate among unvaccinated children.[2]

What happened in the clinical trials?

If we had an unvaccinated group that was like our vaccinated participants, we could estimate how many serious adverse events would have happened to them anyway. Fortunately, we have randomized trials! By comparing reports from the two groups, we see how many 'reactions' were due to the active ingredients, and how many were incidental or from the injection.

Adverse events were reported, without prompting, by 38% receiving the Oxford-AstraZeneca vaccine.[3] Among control participants getting a meningitis vaccine, 28% also reported a side effect, which shows that the specific Covid-19 vaccine only induced around one-third of reported harm. Of more than 24,000 participants in the trials,[4] fewer than 1% reported a serious adverse event and, among these 168 people, slightly more had had the control than the Covid-19 vaccine. Overall, the trial suggested no serious elevation in risk from the Covid-19 vaccine. The Pfizer-BioNTech trials were similar, with more mild or moderate adverse events in the Covid-19 vaccine group, and near-identical numbers of serious adverse events.[5]

The trials led regulators to authorize vaccines for widespread use. However, compared to what will happen after a vaccine is approved for use, clinical trials involve fewer people, focus on short-term outcomes and tend to include healthier individuals. We therefore need to collect 'real-world' **pharmaco-vigilance** data from vaccination programmes.

What happened when the vaccines were rolled out?

In the UK, adverse reactions are recorded using the 'Yellow Card' system, started in 1964 after the thalidomide tragedy. Doctors filled in (you guessed it!) yellow cards* when they suspected a side effect,[6] although the current online system can also be used directly by patients. Of the 22.6 million people who had Oxford-AstraZeneca vaccines up to 28 April 2021,[7] 160,000 submitted reports featuring 597,000 reactions. That is around double the rate for the Pfizer-BioNTech vaccine.

There are large numbers of immediate side effects for all the Covid-19 vaccines, like pain, nausea, fatigue and fever. For the Oxford-AstraZeneca and Pfizer-BioNTech vaccines, there are other reports:† palpitations (4,373), 'feeling jittery' (45), 'screaming' (21), libido increase (five), libido decrease or loss (43), and some unintended pregnancies.

The two vaccines had over 870 anaphylaxis or anaphylactoid reactions. That's around six a day, and why we must sit for 15 minutes after getting jabbed. There were also 722 recorded deaths soon after the Oxford-AstraZeneca jab and 364 after the Pfizer-BioNTech vaccine, which receive thorough examination from regulators.

---

* There have been numerous accounts of why the original system was on yellow cards, such as the colour-blindness of the secretary of the relevant committee, or that the original proposal happened to be typed on yellow paper and this was retained as it was different from other forms and signalled urgency.

† Up to 28 April 2021, there were 14 recorded palpitations after the Moderna and unspecified vaccines. There was one event of jitters after Moderna. At the time, around 100,000 doses of Moderna had been administered.

The Yellow Card system depends on spontaneous reporting of adverse events, which inevitably undercounts the true number. An alternative source of data is from those choosing to use the ZOE app,[8] into which over 600,000 volunteers recorded their side effects following vaccination. Using a pre-specified list, they reported lower rates than those in clinical trials; around two-thirds ticked 'local effects in their arm' and about a quarter had more systemic side effects such as fatigue or fever.

What about blood clots and the Oxford-AstraZeneca vaccine?

In early 2021, there were increasing reports of blood clots in the brain, known as cerebral venous sinus thrombosis (CVST), after the Oxford-AstraZeneca vaccine. This is a serious condition, expected to occur in about one in 75,000 people per year, with a higher rate for younger women.[9] These cases, however, were particularly unusual in that they were also linked to low platelets, which would normally tend to prevent clotting. This phenomenon was later termed VITT (vaccine-induced immune thrombotic thrombocytopenia).*[10] It is challenging to find expected rates of such rare and specific events. By 28 April 2021, the Medicines & Healthcare products Regulatory Agency (MHRA) in the UK had reported 242 such occurrences with 49 deaths.

The problem comes in weighing the potential benefits

---

* This is similar to a rare, and paradoxical, condition in which antibodies made by the patient link to heparin, a potent drug that usually prevents or stops clots, and so trigger the formation of a clot by sticking all the platelets together.

and harms of vaccinating different groups. The benefits of the Covid-19 vaccine increase sharply with age, while risks of serious harm appear to decrease in older people. Figure 23–1 shows an attempt to communicate this balance, as presented by the Deputy Chief Medical Officer, Jonathan Van-Tam, in a public briefing given in April 2021. In that briefing, it was announced that an alternative vaccine should be given to under-30s.

Van-Tam is a trusted communicator and took his time to describe this complex graphic, respecting the audience. Of course, any attempt to summarize all relevant factors is bound to be inadequate.[*]

The risk to young people is portrayed as being around one in 100,000. How do we set such risks in context? Wembley Stadium holds about 90,000 people. If it were crammed with people in their 20s and they all got vaccinated, we would expect one of these serious reactions. Against this, all those people would be largely protected, as would their contacts.

Alternatively, we could compare the incidence to other events. About one in 100,000 sky-dives[11] or surgeries under general anaesthetic ends in death,[12] but these events do not seem comparable to vaccination. Perhaps more similar in nature is the risk of getting a blood clot from the contraceptive pill,[13] which works out at around one in 100,000 *per week*. But such thromboses are usually far less serious than those linked to the Oxford-AstraZeneca vaccine.

Rather than making such comparisons, Figure 23–1

---

[*] Conflict of interest: one of the authors (DS) was part of the team that produced this graphic.

Weighing up the potential benefits and harms of the Oxford–AstraZeneca Covid-19 vaccine

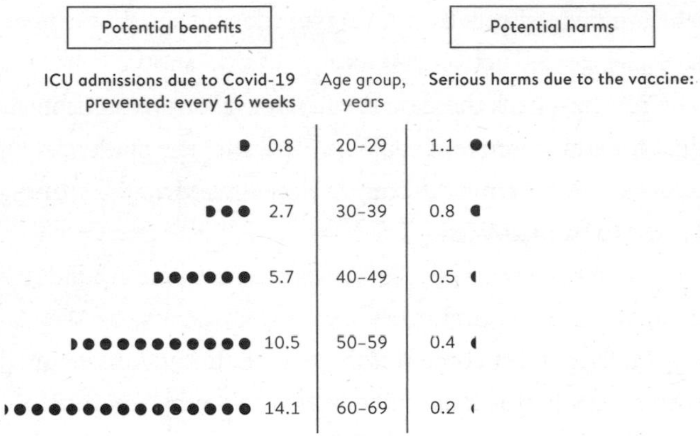

Potential benefits		Potential harms
ICU admissions due to Covid-19 prevented: every 16 weeks	Age group, years	Serious harms due to the vaccine:
● 0.8	20–29	1.1 ●●
●●● 2.7	30–39	0.8 ●
●●●●●● 5.7	40–49	0.5 ●
)●●●●●●●●●● 10.5	50–59	0.4 ●
)●●●●●●●●●●●●●● 14.1	60–69	0.2 ●

Figure 23–1

For 100,000 people with low exposure risk (based on coronavirus incidence of 2 per 10,000: roughly UK in March). Some potential benefits and harms of the Oxford-AstraZeneca vaccine, estimated in early April 2021. ICU admissions are of roughly similar seriousness to the reported blood clots, but unmentioned benefits include prevention of less serious disease and 'long Covid', and crucially the reduction of harm to others by reducing transmission. Less serious harms are also not included. Low-, medium- and high-exposure scenarios were provided.

concentrates on comparing rates of similar events for different age groups , which seems appropriate for such serious post-vaccination side effects.

What side effects are officially reported?

Every approved medical treatment in Europe has an official list of side effects that are reported in an agreed format, using the terms such as 'common' or 'rare' shown in Table 23–1. You can check these on the Patient Information Leaflet (PIL) for any prescribed medicine. Research suggests that we interpret these terms differently to the 'official' definition; in one study, people thought a side effect called 'common' would occur in around 34% of cases, whereas a 1%–10% incidence would be given this label.[14]

As an imperfect comparator, we include the side effects listed on a PIL for a common statin taken by millions of people* to reduce the risk of heart attacks and strokes. In contrast to a one-off vaccination, statins are taken daily, and there is the option of stopping or changing the prescription. On the other hand, statins only help the recipient, while vaccinated people can help others through reduced transmission.

While the European Medicines Agency did not make any recommendations on the Oxford-AstraZeneca vaccine, authorities in many European countries restricted the vaccine to over-60s. Meanwhile, another viral-vector vaccine by Johnson & Johnson was linked to this condition, leading the

---

* Including DS.

Official term	Estimated Frequency	Oxford–AstraZeneca vaccine	Pfizer–BioNTech vaccine	Atorvastatin
Very common	More than 10% (1 in 10)	Temporary pain and tenderness, headache, chills, nausea	Temporary pain and tenderness, headache, chills, fever, joint pain	
Common	1% to 10% (1 in 100 to 1 in 10)	Swelling and redness at injection site, fever, vomiting, diarrhoea, flu-like symptoms	Redness at injection site, nausea, vomiting	Muscle pain, headache, nausea
Uncommon	0.1% to 1% (1 in 1,000 to 1 in 100)	Enlarged lymph nodes, dizziness, sweating, rash	Enlarged lymph nodes, feeling unwell, arm pain	Anorexia, nightmares, blurred vision, rash
Rare	0.01% to 0.1% (1 in 10,000 to 1 in 1,000)		Temporary one-sided facial drooping	Serious allergic reaction or muscle injury (rhabdomyolysis)
Very rare	Less than 0.01% (< 1 in 10,000)	Thrombosis with thrombocytopenia		Liver disease, hearing loss

US Food and Drug Administration to pause its roll-out in April 2021.[16]

So far, these vaccines have shown themselves to be relatively safe for such an effective intervention. Perhaps the most surprising thing is that we have not heard far more stories of adverse effects. But cases of young, healthy people being harmed by vaccination rightly have a strong emotional impact, even though such serious adverse events are extremely rare.

[Facing page] Table 23–1
Some of the side-effect information for Covid-19 vaccines, as listed by the MHRA in April 2021.[15] Severe allergic reactions can occur with both vaccines but are not given a frequency. Atorvastatin side effects are taken from the patient information leaflet (PIL). Reported events in the PIL could still be incidental.

Who has been getting the vaccines?

Having developed effective and safe vaccines, the crucial question is: who gets the vaccines first?

There are two general strategies when there is a lot of virus circulating: vaccinate people who spread the virus or protect the vulnerable. When vaccination priorities were being set near the end of 2020, it was uncertain to what extent vaccines curtailed transmission.[1] The Joint Committee on Vaccination and Immunisation (JCVI)[2] chose the primary aim of reducing deaths and illness in vulnerable groups.[3]

The question then became statistical: who is most at risk of catching and then dying from Covid-19? As we saw in Chapter 13, two major independent studies, QCovid[4] and OpenSAFELY,[5] concluded that age is the dominant risk factor. Based on these analyses, the JCVI defined nine priority groups down to those aged 50 or over,[6] as shown in Table 24–1 with estimated numbers in the UK,[7] and first doses by 30 April 2021, estimated from OpenSAFELY.[8]

These nine top-priority groups accounted for about 99% of all deaths related to Covid-19, but the same prioritization by age would be appropriate if minimizing years of life lost rather than simply mortality. This risk ranking was

	Group	Rough numbers in UK (millions)	Estimated % with first dose (by 30 April 2021)
1	Care home residents.	0.3	96%
	Care home carers.	0.5	-
2	Those aged 80 or over	3.3	96%
	Front-line healthcare workers	3.8	-
3	All those of 75–79 years of age	2.3	96%
4	All those of 70–74 years of age.	3.2	96%
	Clinically extremely vulnerable individuals under 70	1.2	87%
5	All those of 65–69 years of age	2.9	93%
6	All those aged 16–64 with underlying health conditions	7.3	81%
7	All those of 60–64 years of age	1.8	90%
8	All those of 55–59 years of age	2.4	88%
9	All those of 50–54 years of age	2.8	85%
	Total Priority Groups	32	
	Rest of adult population	21	

Table 24–1
Nine priority groups identified by the JCVI, with approximate numbers in the UK. Clinically extremely vulnerable people are those with severe health conditions, who had been shielding since the start of the pandemic. The one-dose-vaccinated proportion for 70 to 79-year-olds is applied to both age sub-groups.[*]

[*] NHS England used 2019 population estimates as denominators, which can be too low and result in some older groups apparently having vaccination rates greater than 100%.

approximate – for example, no account is taken of men being at higher risk than women.

In the UK there was a clear prioritization, with little capacity for 'gaming' or jumping the queue: the Queen received her vaccine on 9 January 2021, while the Duchess of Cambridge had to wait her turn until 28 May when the roll-out included her age-group (35–39).

Were higher-risk occupations prioritized?

We've seen in Chapter 13 that some public-facing occupations, such as care workers and bus drivers, faced higher relative risks from Covid-19. There was also strong pressure for vaccination of teachers before reopening schools. But the only prioritized occupational groups were those most likely to infect vulnerable people, and further recommendations beyond the nine priority groups were based solely on age.[9]

In the US, the prioritization of the Centers for Disease Control and Prevention was somewhat different.[10] The first vaccines went to health-care workers and residents of long-term care facilities, while in 'Phase 1b', vaccines went to those aged 75 and older and a wide range of front-line essential workers including police officers and teachers.

Who has been taking the vaccine?

High rates of overall vaccine coverage shown in Table 24–1 obscure some important disparities. The OpenSAFELY data show that 91% of those aged 60–64 had received their first jab by 26 May 2021, but that share fell to 68% among Black people, and 77% among people with mixed ethnicity.

Hesitancy to have the vaccine will play a part in lowering

coverage, and a qualitative ONS study,[11] based on 50 in-depth interviews in February–March 2021, revealed that concerns about the vaccine included safety, particularly due to its rapid development: 'I feel like it's too early. I don't feel enough time or research has passed. I don't know what the effects from the vaccine will be after five, 10 or 15 years from now.' Some younger people fear the vaccine's effects on fertility, and others feel they don't need it anyway. There is some suspicion of its being derived from a chimpanzee virus or cells from a human foetus, as well as general distrust of the pharmaceutical industry and government. Unfortunately, as we saw in Chapter 20, there has been extensive misinformation. 'In real life I've heard it's working and it's fine. On the Internet I've heard loads of people have died from the vaccine, so there's real life and online.'

How many people have antibodies to the virus?

We've seen in Chapter 7 how antibody data is collected as part of the ONS Covid-19 Infection Survey; in 2020 this gave an idea of the impact of the virus, but in 2021 antibodies could be due to either previous infection *or* vaccination.

[Following pages] Figure 24–1
Modelled proportion of people testing positive for antibodies in blood samples for different age groups between December 2020 and April 2021, together with the proportion receiving one and two doses of the vaccine.

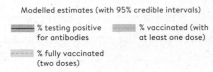

Modelled estimates (with 95% credible intervals)

— % testing positive for antibodies

— % vaccinated (with at least one dose)

----- % fully vaccinated (two doses)

Source: Office for National Statistics – Covid-19 infection survey

In England, antibody positivity has risen sharply in older age groups

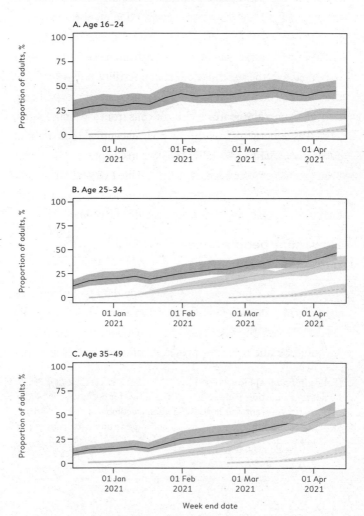

A. Age 16–24

B. Age 25–34

C. Age 35–49

Week end date

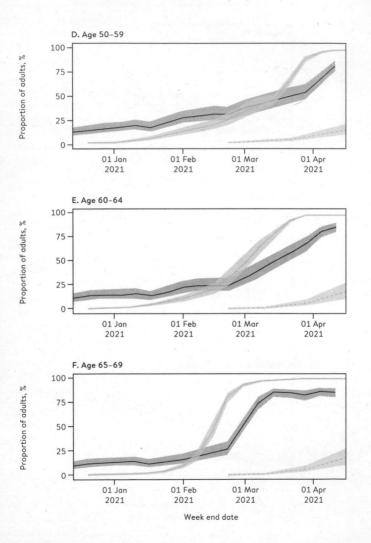

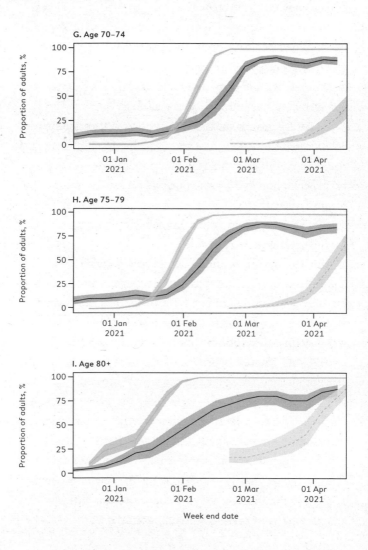

Figure 24–1 shows the modelled estimates of the proportion of each age group in England that would test positive for antibodies, indicating the changes during the vaccine roll-out.[12]

Figure 24–1 shows that those aged 16–24 were the most likely to test positive for antibodies before the start of the vaccination programme, and by April 2021 nearly half had antibodies: the minority due to vaccination. The virus had spread extensively through young adults.

Older age groups started at lower levels of antibodies developed after infection, but then vaccination led to a rapid rise. There is an inevitable lag of around two weeks between first vaccination and testing positive for antibodies, but the proportion with antibodies does not fully rise to meet the level of those receiving their first jab, emphasizing the need for full vaccination.

Having antibodies after a symptomatic infection or vaccination does not confer complete or necessarily enduring immunity, and knowing how antibodies rise (and fall) after vaccination is vital to help plan for booster jabs. As more people develop antibodies – even with incomplete protection – immunity grows, the population becomes less susceptible, and the spread of the virus is slowed.

Once the goals of a vaccine programme are set, statistics can help answer questions of equitable priority. The lower vaccine coverage in certain ethnic groups, which we know tend to be of higher risk, is concerning for the future protection of some communities. But this does not negate the success and popularity of the vaccine roll-out in the UK.

How far apart should the vaccines be given?

The UK initially gave second doses of Covid-19 vaccines 12 weeks after the first dose, longer than the three-week gap used as a target in the Pfizer-BioNTech randomized controlled trial and by countries elsewhere. What was the reasoning behind what *The Washington Post* described as 'one big, high-stakes science experiment'?[1]

The stated goal of the vaccination programme was to save lives. Each dose should reduce the marginal risk of death. There are limited doses of vaccines, and longer dosing intervals mean that more people are protected, faster. This is an **optimization problem** against supply constraints, time and a deadly virus, and mathematical modelling suggested – given the first dose provided reasonable efficacy – that more lives would be saved by lengthening that gap.[2]

Figure 25–1 shows that at the start of March 2021, jabs were averaging around 350,000 a day and were nearly all first doses. People started coming to the end of their 12-week gap and needed their second doses. The strategy worked: by 17 February 2021, around 17 million vaccine doses had been given in the UK.[3] Over 16 million had received their first

After an initial period of first doses, UK focus shifted to second doses in March 2021

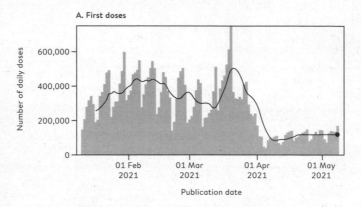

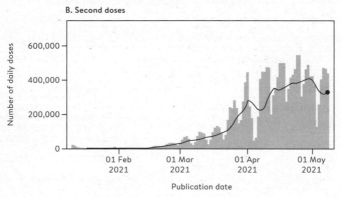

Figure 25–1

Seven-day rolling average of UK first- and second-dose vaccinations, by publication date.

Source: Public Health England Covid-19 dashboard data download

dose; had there been a three-week interval, only around 10 million would have had any vaccine.

What protection does a single dose provide?

If the delayed-second-dose strategy is to save lives, there needs to be good protection in the gap between the first ('priming') and second ('boosting') doses, which can be up to three months. Fortunately, in the clinical trials that estimated efficacy, most protection came from the first dose, but second doses provided enhanced and enduring immunity.[4] A small pre-print study of Maryland health-care workers found that messenger RNA vaccines had much bigger antibody responses in those with a past SARS-CoV-2 infection, with earlier infections from the virus acting like a priming dose from a vaccine.[5]

A clear concern is whether a longer dosing interval harms overall effectiveness, but this has not been found for other vaccines and, for biological reasons, was judged unlikely for virus-vectored ones. Andrew Pollard, head of the Oxford Vaccine Group, said: 'Generally, a longer gap between vaccine doses leads to a better immune response, with the second dose causing a better boost.'[6] The summary was: 'The immune system remembers the first dose and will respond whether the later dose is at three weeks or three months.'

For the Oxford-AstraZeneca vaccine, exploratory analysis indicated there was higher efficacy from a longer dosing interval;[7] with two standard doses and a dosing interval of less than six weeks, researchers reported trial efficacy against symptomatic Covid-19 of 55% (33%–70%). For a prime-boost interval of more than 12 weeks, that efficacy rose to 81% (60%–91%).

A further concern is whether the immunity from one dose substantially wanes across the 12 weeks. Some decline in antibodies was found in experimental work on the Pfizer-BioNTech vaccine,[8] while the ONS Covid-19 Infection Survey found a small drop in those testing positive with antibodies while specific age groups were 'between vaccines'.[9] In contrast, Public Health England vaccine-effectiveness studies estimated an improvement with time after the first dose.[10] A pre-print analysis of 172 people aged 80 or over found a similar pattern for the Pfizer-BioNTech vaccine.[11]

UK institutions made bold decisions in the vaccination programme: approval of the Oxford-AstraZeneca vaccine in older people, despite low numbers of Covid-19 cases in trial participants; rigorous prioritization to save lives; and increasing the gap between doses to maximize protection. But if the underlying conditions change, then the optimal strategy also evolves. So, in the light of evidence that the new Delta (B.1.617.2) variant reduced the effectiveness of a single dose, on 21 May the JCVI recommended accelerating second doses, and reducing the gap between doses for higher-risk groups 1–9 from 12 weeks to eight weeks.

In this global pandemic, both science and interventions are done at speed. Decisions must be made using imperfect data and limited background knowledge, in the face of intractable uncertainty.

Looking Forwards and Back

How good are the projections from epidemic models?

From the start of the pandemic, epidemiological models have been a source of continuing controversy, blamed for fear-mongering and inaccuracy. How well have they done?

Epidemiology is the study of public health outcomes across populations,[1] and an important tool is to try to distil problems down to their essence, described in mathematical terms: this is called a model. Models have numerous uses, including:

- making predictions or projections, based on a range of assumptions – see this chapter
- understanding the virus and epidemic – see Chapter 13
- estimating the effects of the anti-transmission measures – see Chapter 16
- estimating the effectiveness of vaccines – see Chapter 22
- establishing priorities for resources such as vaccines – see Chapter 24.

The most commonly used models can be termed **mechanistic,** since they try to construct a simplified version of the actual mechanism by which a virus spreads through the population. The most basic type are SIR models (Figure 26–1), in which people are in one of three 'compartments':

- *susceptible*: they can catch the disease from others
- *infected*: they have the disease and may pass it to others
- *recovered (or removed)*: they have had the disease and can no longer catch it.*

There are many sources of uncertainty in modelling. First, there is the unavoidable unpredictability of the future, which is often handled by simulating the possible outcomes for huge numbers of individuals. Second, there is uncertainty about underlying assumptions, such as the appropriate value of the current reproduction number R_t, (the average number of people that a case infects); this leads to sensitivity analysis, exploring differing assumptions. Finally, there is the uncertainty due to the inevitable inadequacy in modelling reality. Every model is a simplification – it is a map, not the territory. That is why it helps to have multiple independent teams constructing models.

A famous analysis was published by Professor Neil Ferguson's team at Imperial College London on 16 March 2020,[2] credited with provoking the full lockdown announced for 23 March. Their model is more complex than the simple SIR structure, breaking contacts into areas such as households

---

* There are many variants of this simple design. For deadly diseases, modellers create a SIRD model with a deceased state. There may be another category – exposed – added to such models, which represents a non-infectious incubation period, resulting in a SEIR model. Another version is that there is no immunity granted by infection, which means people revert to being susceptible after infection, forming a SIS compartmental model.

The SIR model is a simple way of putting people into compartments

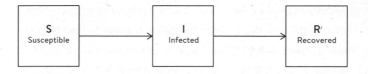

Figure 26-1
The SIR model, with compartments that people move through, from susceptible to infectious to recovered.

and workplaces, and making assumptions on the viral incubation period, infectiousness, length of hospital stays and more.

The model considers the impacts of different non-pharmaceutical interventions on what we expect to happen to cases, hospitalizations and deaths, all estimated by simulating the future lives of thousands of imaginary individuals: such **stochastic** modelling is very computer-intensive. The reproduction number was assumed to be 2.4, although values between 2.0 and 2.6 were tried.

They first looked at the consequences of 'the (unlikely) absence of any control measures or spontaneous changes in individual behaviour', projecting 510,000 deaths in Great Britain over two years, and 2.2 million in the US. Unfortunately, it has been repeatedly claimed that the model estimated there would be half a million deaths.* That was not a prediction, but a projection under the implausible scenario where the virus spreads and nobody does anything about it.

Their model explored a wide range of scenarios, and suggested a large impact from mitigation policies. With case isolation, home quarantine, social distancing and school and university closure, the highest projection for deaths in Great Britain was projected to be 48,000 over two years, which has turned out to be rather optimistic. In contrast, their projections for intensive-care usage tended to be too high.

Alternative ways of modelling do not simulate dynamic diseases, but instead use ideas of **curve-fitting** to series of

---

* For example, *The Washington Post* reported: 'Imperial College scientist who predicted 500K coronavirus deaths in UK adjusts figure to 20K or fewer.'

data points such as cases or deaths, and then project that curve forwards in time. It is like seeing the initial arc of a thrown ball and estimating how high and far that ball goes. Like a thrown ball, these models assume conditions do not change, and this has led to some overconfident and erroneous forecasts.[3]

The University of Washington's Institute for Health Metrics (IHME) model suggested in early May 2020 that California would have no Covid-19 deaths by the end of that month.[4] The California Department of Public Health subsequently reported over 49,000 Covid-19 deaths after May 2020.[5]

How good were projections made in July 2020?

Planning for emergencies has traditionally focused on the construction of 'reasonable worst-case scenarios' (RWCS), based on the idea of 'plan for the worst, hope for the best', and so adopting deliberately pessimistic assumptions. In July 2020, the SAGE committee considered an RWCS for the nine months from 1 July 2020 to 31 March 2021, summarized in Table 26–1, with the subsequent actual outcomes.[6]

In general, the scenario was reasonably prescient, although it placed the peak of the second wave somewhat later than subsequently occurred. Indeed, reality turned out worse than the 'worst-case scenario', with more reported deaths and higher peak hospital occupancy. At that time there was no certainty that vaccines would be available, although the new Alpha (B.1.1.7) variant had not started to make an impact.

Perhaps a low point for the public perception of modelling

Measure	Reasonable Worst-Case Scenario stated in July 2020	Actual value
Number of Covid-19 deaths	85,000	96,000
Peak daily Covid-19 deaths	800 (late February 2021)	1,500 (mid-January 2021)
Covid-19 hospitalisations	356,000	331,000
Peak daily hospital (non-ICU) occupancy	25,000 (late February 2021)	39,000 (mid-January 2021)
Peak daily ICU occupancy	6,000 (late Mar 2021)	

Table 26–1
UK projections made in July 2020 under a reasonable worst-case scenario (RWCS) for outcomes between 1 July 2020 and 31 March 2021, compared with what actually happened (rounded to the nearest thousand). Covid-19 deaths are from the ONS. Hospitalizations and occupancy refer to the 'patients admitted to hospital' and 'patients in hospital' measures.

occurred at the end of October 2020, when some projections were leaked that showed a possible future peak of 4,000 deaths a day. But these model outputs were never meant to be released, and had already been revised downwards before the leak. Despite that, they formed part of the public briefing and presentations to parliament, leading to criticism by the statistics watchdog: the UK Statistics Authority said, 'full transparency of data used to inform decisions is vital to public understanding and public confidence'.[7]

The 'roadmap' for release from lockdown announced on 22 February 2021 was informed by models from multiple independent teams,[8] focusing on a 'central estimate' as well as more pessimistic scenarios.[9] Even cautious strategies were projected to lead to more than 50,000 deaths by June 2022 (with a 95% uncertainty interval of 33,000–81,000), and nearly double that with earlier relaxation, which will have influenced the apparent caution in the roadmap. These projections were regularly revised in the light of new evidence on variants, vaccine coverage and effectiveness, and will continue to change.

How good is human judgement?

Although based on numerous judgements, models offer some degree of objectivity when making predictions. How do they compare with purely subjective judgements about what might happen?

In early April 2020, DS and colleagues surveyed 140 UK experts and over 2,000 UK laypersons, asking them to make four quantitative predictions about the impact of Covid-19 on the UK by the end of 2020.[10] The experts gave a median estimate of the number of Covid-19 deaths as 30,000, while non-experts said 20,000; in reality, on 31 December 2020 the UK reported a total of 76,000 Covid-19 deaths. The respondents also provided an interval in which they were 75% confident the true value would lie, but the recorded value was contained in only 36% of the experts' intervals and only 10% of the non-experts'. Humans were both too optimistic and too sure of themselves – a common finding.*

It is worth remembering two classic quotes: 'predictions are difficult, especially about the future', and 'all models are wrong, but some are useful'.[11] Epidemic models are always full of uncertainty, which flows from their simplified structure, their assumptions and data inputs and the unpredictability of real life. Provided we view these models as tools for our understanding, they can still be useful.

---

* On 16 March 2020, DS wrote down (although did not say publicly) that he was 65% confident there would be between 5,000 and 15,000 deaths from Covid-19 in the UK, like a moderate flu season, and gave only a 10% chance to there being more than 15,000 deaths. He displayed chronic optimism.

What is going to happen in the future?

There are many forking paths to possible futures, with much that is unknown and unknowable. In terms of the virus, we can identify three broad scenarios for countries:[1]

- **Endemic:** The SARS-CoV-2 virus becomes endemic, at low levels with seasonal cycles. Harms depend on overall infections and immunity, as well as effective treatments and vaccinations. This was the fate of the 2009 H1N1 influenza virus,[2] becoming part of the influenza herd. Like influenza, SARS-CoV-2 may become an acceptable risk to society, although even in 'good' years there could be thousands of deaths in large countries. Booster vaccines will be updated for the latest variants.

- **Containment:** Testing, tracing and isolation programmes help contain the SARS-CoV-2 virus. There can be localized flaring and infections. It takes time for containment to erode the virus, as it did with the original SARS virus.[3]

- **Elimination:** The number of infections is reduced to essentially zero for a sustained period. Countries then remain at risk of importation and may need to retain strict border controls.

Countries are not independent of each other. Will Covid-19 become more politicized, with uncoordinated responses, closed borders and stoked tensions? Will countries share vaccines and expertise? The future is likely to be mixed.

What about the UK? As we write this sentence in May 2021, modelling had suggested there would be an 'exit wave',[4] with Covid-19 surging as people mixed more and went back to school and work. Real-world data allowed modellers to update those assumptions, permitting more optimism,[5] but then the Delta (B.1.617.2) variant intruded. There is great uncertainty about the next few months as the virus spreads primarily among younger people, with a wide range of outcomes compatible with the current evidence.

In the longer term, there could be an exuberant embrace of social activity, but some people may remain deeply anxious about returning to normal life, and they will be the ones we do not see. There are likely to be many memorial events to those whose deaths could not be marked appropriately at the time. There is also likely to be a delayed impact on foregone medical investigations and treatments, and long-term effects on employment and the educational prospects of young people.

As in wars, the young will pay the price of protecting those who are more vulnerable.

Postscript

The last year has been a story of strife, suffering, science and statistics. News broadcasts and articles have been awash with numbers: cases, R, daily deaths, vaccine efficacy and more.

Statistics is the art of learning from data. Every number has been a sharp summary of human experience. Millions have died. Many more have gone through hospital doors. As well as the huge debt we owe to health-care and essential workers, we should also thank statisticians and analysts in governments, public health agencies and other organizations for their service under severe circumstances.

It is natural that people will want to review how their countries reacted to the pandemic, and we leave it to future inquiries to examine questions about pandemic preparedness, the role of scientific advice, the protection of the vulnerable in care homes, the pressures on health-care staff, the timing and effectiveness of interventions, the balances between national and local responses, public procurement, vaccine strategy and much more. All these issues will require careful attention to data, and we hope this book will contribute to an improved discussion.

There are clearly many lessons that can be drawn from the pandemic, but as statisticians we shall focus on the ones concerned with data. Fortunately, the Royal Statistical Society has produced a list of ten statistical lessons from the UK's experience:[1]

1. **Invest in public health data**

   Good public health data are essential for understanding the pandemic, but insights are limited due to inadequate and fragmented resources. More investment is needed both in systems and in people.

2. **Publish the evidence**

   People have been asked to make huge sacrifices based on uncertain and evolving evidence. Citizens deserve clarity about the basis of the decisions that affect them, underpinned by coherent summaries and available datasets.

3. **Be clear and open about the data**

   Unless there are overwhelming contradictory reasons, data should be transparent and publicly available. The ONS and Public Health England have both innovated in terms of their openness, but it can be difficult to navigate the analyses produced by different organizations.

4. **Challenge the misuse of statistics**

   The Office for Statistics Regulation has held ministers to account, but its role for non-departmental statistics is unclear. Greater data transparency will assist organizations such as Full Fact and the Science Media Centre to provide more effective challenges.

5. **The media need to recognize their responsibilities**

   The statistical literacy of journalists seems to have improved, but news organizations can still treat the pandemic as a primarily political story, rather than calling upon the experience of health and science journalists.

6. **Build decision-makers' statistical skills**
   Statistical thinking is vital in a pandemic. Politicians, civil servants and scientists must understand the strengths and limitations of the available data and statistics, and people with established statistical skills need to be at the 'top table' when making decisions.

7. **Maintain an effective infectious disease surveillance system**
   Timeliness of statistics matters for public health. A real-time public health surveillance system should be ready for the next health emergency.

8. **Improve scrutiny of diagnostic testing**
   Vaccine and pharmaceutical evaluations follow rigorous steps, which should also be applied to diagnostic testing. Manufacturers should release their studies in sufficient detail so that their marketing claims can be examined.

9. **Health-care data remain incomplete without social-care data**
   There has been a lack of data on social care in England, including even basic counts of residents. That paucity of data made it difficult to understand the causes of the impact on care homes.

10. **Put evaluation at the heart of policy**
    Evaluating treatments in the RECOVERY trials has been a huge success, and it is extraordinary that so much money has been spent on interventions such as NHS Test and Trace with little idea of its impact. A scientific

approach, including experimentation, can help improve public policy.

Whatever the future brings, we personally hope that the extraordinary focus on statistics over the pandemic will have raised the interest of government, the media and the public in the proper use of data in our daily lives. This would, at least, mean one positive benefit from the last year.

Glossary

Absolute risk: the proportion of people in a defined group who experience an event of interest within a specified period.

Adverse events: a medical problem occurring during drug treatments or other therapies. Adverse events may be mild, moderate or severe, and can have causes other than the administered drug or therapy.

Age-standardized mortality rate: a calculation which uses age-specific mortality rates (such as the proportion of people aged 75–79 who died) and derives an overall rate as a weighted average. The weights in this average are from a standard population, like the '2013 European Standard Population'. Comparisons based on this standardization then account for differing population size and age structure.

All-cause mortality: registered deaths from any cause in a specific period.

Attack rate: the proportion of people that contract a disease in a specified period. This is the absolute risk of contracting a disease.

Basic reproduction number: the average number of secondary infections from a single, typical infection in a completely susceptible population. This dimensionless number is affected

by the transmissibility of the virus, average contacts, and the
duration of infectiousness.

Bayes' Theorem: a rule of probability that shows how evidence
A updates prior beliefs of an event B to produce 'posterior'
beliefs $P(B|A)$, meaning the probability of B given A. This is
through the formula:

$$P(B|A) = \frac{P(A|B)\ P(B)}{P(A)}$$

This is easy to prove, since the multiplication rule of
probability and the symmetry of two events occurring at
once means:

$$P(B|A)\ P(A) = (A \text{ and } B) = P(B \text{ and } A) = P(A|B)\ P(B)$$

Dividing each side by $P(A)$ gives the formula.

Clinical trial phases: a Phase I trial is the first small test on
humans. The main aims in Phase I are to ensure the treatment
presents no major safety issues and gather preliminary
evidence of restorative or preventative value. Phase II trials
are larger, aiming to establish rough estimates in efficacy and
appropriate dosing regimens. Phase III trials are even larger,
often involving thousands of volunteers. The objectives are
demonstrating safety and efficacy, confirming effective doses,
identifying side effects and risks, and comparing results
against existing treatments. Phase IV studies comprise post-
approval surveillance, so-called pharmaco-vigilance.

Collider bias: a collider is causally influenced by two or more
variables. Controlling on a collider variable, through design
or analysis, can induce distorted associations between other
variables.

GLOSSARY

Confidence interval: an estimated interval within which an unknown parameter may plausibly lie. Based on the observed data, a 95% confidence interval for µ is an interval whose lower limit L(x) and upper limit U(x) has the property that, before observing the data, there is a 95% probability that the random interval (L(x), U(x)) contains µ. The Central Limit Theorem, combined with the knowledge that close to 95% of a normal distribution lies between the mean ± two standard deviations, means a common approximation for a 95% confidence interval ± two standard errors.

Confounder: a variable which is associated with both a response and a predictor, and which may explain some of the apparent relationship. For example, the height and weight of children are strongly correlated, but much of this association is explained by their age.

Credible interval: an interval within which a parameter (treated as a random variable in Bayesian analysis) falls within a given probability. Credible intervals are not unique, and there are many ways to choose such intervals. For distributions with a single mode, suitable credible intervals include: choosing values of highest probability density, equal-tailed intervals containing the median, or intervals centred around the mean.

Crude mortality rate: the number of registered deaths in a specific period, expressed as a proportion of the population.

Curve-fitting: the process of constructing a mathematical function which suits data points. That can involve interpolation between data points and smoothing.

Cycle threshold: the cycle number at which the fluorescence generated within a reaction crosses a threshold representing background fluorescence. It is the first cycle at which the gene of interest is detected.

Effective reproduction number: the average number of second cases per infectious case, in a population containing both susceptible and non-susceptible people. Prior infections and vaccinations can make people non-susceptible to the disease, reducing the susceptible population.

Excess deaths: the number of deaths in a specific period minus a baseline value for deaths. The baseline value could represent the average deaths over the past five years or be a model of expected deaths.

Exponential growth: a process which increases a quantity over time, in multiples. For example, a bacterium doubles in time: splitting in two, then four, then eight, then 16, and so on. This term does not mean 'fast': your money in a low-interest savings account is growing exponentially. In mathematical terms, exponential growth looks like:

$$x_t = x_0 \, (1 + r)^t$$

Taking logarithms gives

$$\log x_t = \log x_0 + t \log (1 + r),$$

which is linear in time.

Genomic sequencing: the process of determining the whole (or nearly whole) genetic sequence of an organism's genome at a single time. This sequencing helps epidemiologists and public health researchers understand how the virus is spreading and changing.

Hazard ratio: when analysing survival times, the relative risk, associated with an exposure, of suffering an event in a fixed period. A Cox regression is a form of multiple regression when the response variable is a survival time, and the coefficients correspond to the logarithm of hazard ratios.

Infection fatality rate (IFR): the proportion of those infected who died from that infection.

Logarithmic scale: the logarithm to base 10 of a positive number x is denoted by $y = \log_{10}x$, or equivalently $x = 10^y$. In statistical analysis and mathematical textbooks, $\log x$ generally denotes the natural logarithm $y = \log_e x$, where e is the exponential constant (or Euler's number), roughly equal to 2.718.

Margins of sampling error: after a survey, analysts often calculate 95% confidence intervals, approximately the mean ± two standard errors. Those two standard errors are often called the margin of error, reflecting errors in survey estimates due to sampling. For a simple random sample of 1,000 people, the margin of sampling error around a true value of 50% (where errors are maximized) is ± three percentage points.

Matched control study: a study design where cases (such as vaccinated people) are matched to controls (such as unvaccinated people) based upon some characteristics. The idea is to match upon potential confounding variables and reduce those biases.

Mean (of a sample): suppose we have a set of n data points. Their sample mean is the sum of the data points divided by n. In mathematical formula, that is:

$$\overline{x} = \frac{1}{n} \sum_{i=1}^{n} x_i$$

If our sample were 3, 2, 1, 0, 1, then the sample mean is $(3 + 2 + 1 + 0 + 1)/5 = 1.4$.

Mechanistic: a type of model where mathematical formulae describe physical, biological or technical processes. For example, we could construct a mechanistic model of a forest fire. Each tree burns for one step in time, setting every surrounding tree alight. The starting conditions then uniquely determine the outcome of this mechanistic model.

Median (of a sample): the value midway along the ordered set of data points. If n is odd, then the sample median is the middle value of an ordered set. If n is even, then the median is the average of the two middle points.

Mode (of a sample): the most common value in a set of data. In a population distribution, the mode is the response with the highest probability of occurring.

Mortality displacement: a phenomenon where a period of excess deaths (where deaths are higher than expectations) is followed by deficit deaths (where deaths are under expectations). Another name is 'harvesting'. Mortality displacement can follow environmental events, such as heatwaves or cold snaps. Deaths can also be displaced forwards in time, say through a mild winter or low seasonal flu.

Optimization problem: a mathematical problem where the goal is to select the best choice within constraints, from a set of possible alternatives. Such problems often involve maximization or minimization of functions from a permitted set of input values.

Pharmaco-vigilance: the practice of monitoring the effects of drugs after being licensed for use. A common goal is the detection, understanding and prevention of adverse events from medicines.

Population fatality rate (PFR): the proportion of a total population that have died from a disease.

Positivity: the proportion of tests (or tested people) which return a positive result within a specified period.

Predictive values: the positive predictive value is the probability that a person with a positive test has the disease. The negative predictive value is the chance that someone with a negative result does not have the disease.

Prospective cohort study: when a set of individuals are identified, background factors are measured, and then they are followed up and relevant outcomes observed.

Randomized control trial (RCT): an experimental design in which people or other units being tested are randomly allocated to different interventions, thus ensuring, up to the play of chance, that the groups are balanced in both known and unknown background factors. If the groups show subsequent substantial differences in outcome, then either the effect must be due to the intervention or a surprising event has occurred.

Recall error: errors when survey respondents are asked to remember past events or experiences. Participants may completely forget something happened or misremember parts of their experience.

Relative risk: if the absolute risk among people who are exposed to something of interest is p, and the absolute risk among people who are not exposed is q, then the relative risk is p/q.

RNA: ribonucleic acid. This is like DNA, but only has a single strand. There are many types of RNA, of which the three well-studied types are messenger RNA (mRNA), transfer RNA (tRNA) and ribosomal RNA (rRNA), present in all organisms.

Rolling average: a calculation to analyse data points through creating a series of different averages, which represent different subsets of the full set, say over a week centred on the day of interest. This is useful for time series data to smooth out fluctuations, highlighting trends.

Sample survey: a collected subset of a population, used to estimate characteristics of the overall population. A common example is political polling, which uses surveys to estimate how people intend to vote in an upcoming election (among other questions).

Secondary attack rate (SAR): the proportion of an infected person's contacts (such as in the household or close contacts) who also become infected. The initial infected person is often called the index case.

Sensitivity: the proportion of 'positive' cases that are correctly identified by a classifier or test. This is often termed the true-positive rate. One minus sensitivity is also known as the observed Type II error or false-negative rate.

Seroreversion: the decrease over time in specific antibody levels so they measure below the detection threshold of a test. It can be transient, meaning antibody levels fluctuate between being detected and not detected.

Social desirability bias: the tendency of some survey respondents to answer questions in a way they deem would be acceptable to others, rather than give their 'true' answer. People may over-report socially desirable attitudes and behaviours (like voting) and under-report undesirable ones (such as taking illicit drugs).

Specificity: the proportion of 'negative' cases that are correctly identified by a classifier or test. One minus specificity is the observed Type I error, or false-positive rate.

Statistical model: a mathematical representation, containing unknown parameters, of the probability of a set of random variables.

Stochastic: the process can be well described by a probability distribution. In statistical modelling, it means the outcomes of the modelling process are probabilistic, and so analysts can then run these models many times, to estimate the uncertainty in those outcomes.

Vaccine effectiveness: in vaccine deployment programmes, studies can estimate the reduction in disease among vaccinated people compared to unvaccinated people. Due to how large these programmes are, vaccine effectiveness studies can estimate the reduction in rare outcomes, such as hospitalization and death.

Vaccine efficacy: in a clinical trial, the reduction in disease among vaccinated participants compared to the control group.

Weighting (in surveys): weights are statistical adjustments made to survey data, seeking to improve the accuracy of survey estimates. There are different kinds of survey weights: adjusting for selection probabilities, non-response, and mirroring population distributions.

Wild-type SARS-CoV-2: a form of the virus containing no major mutations.

Notes

CHAPTER 1: INTRODUCTION

1. https://coronavirus.data.gov.uk/
2. https://covidtracking.com/
3. https://www.penguin.co.uk/books/195/195518/the-signal-and-the-noise/9780141975658.html
4. https://ourworldindata.org/explorers/coronavirus-data-explorer
5. https://velvetgloveironfist.blogspot.com/2021/02/covid-19-mythbuster.html
   https://fullfact.org/health/can-we-believe-lockdown-sceptics/
   https://www.covidfaq.co/

CHAPTER 2: HOW DID THE PANDEMIC DEVELOP?

1. https://www.who.int/news/item/29-06-2020-Covidtimeline
2. https://promedmail.org/promed-post/?id=6864153%20#Covid19
3. https://virological.org/t/novel-2019-coronavirus-genome/319
4. https://www.who.int/publications/i/item/10665-330374?sequence=1&isAllowed=y
5. https://news.sky.com/story/Covid-19-its-been-a-year-since-cases-were-reported-in-the-uk-12201509
6. https://ourworldindata.org/Covid-deaths
7. https://coronavirus.data.gov.uk/details/cases
8. https://www.health.org.uk/news-and-comment/charts-and-infographics/Covid-19-policy-tracker
9. https://www.gov.uk/government/publications/budget-2020-documents
10. https://www.bbc.co.uk/news/uk-politics-56361599

11. https://www.who.int/docs/default-source/coronaviruse/situation-reports/20200316-sitrep-56-Covid-19.pdf?sfvrsn=9fda7db2_6

12. https://www.imperial.ac.uk/media/imperial-college/medicine/sph/ide/gida-fellowships/Imperial-College-Covid19-NPI-modelling-16-03-2020.pdf

13. https://www.gov.uk/government/speeches/pm-address-to-the-nation-on-coronavirus-23-march-2020

14. https://news.sky.com/story/covid-19-daughter-of-first-uk-victim-questions-when-coronavirus-arrived-in-the-country-12203040

15. https://ourworldindata.org/Covid-models

16. https://www.alumni.ox.ac.uk/article/revealed-how-Covid-19-came-into-the-uk

17. https://www.bbc.co.uk/sport/football/52399569

18. https://www.ncbi.nlm.nih.gov/pmc/articles/PMC7451011/

19. https://www.bbc.co.uk/sport/football/51815623

20. https://assets.publishing.service.gov.uk/government/uploads/system/uploads/attachment_data/file/986168/Weekly_Flu_and_Covid-19_report_w19.pdf

21. https://www.bmj.com/content/371/bmj.m4906

22. https://www.gov.uk/government/publications/Covid-19-response-spring-2021/Covid-19-response-spring-2021-summary

---

CHAPTER 3: HOW INFECTIOUS IS SARS-COV-2?

1. https://www.ncbi.nlm.nih.gov/pmc/articles/PMC7224694/

2. https://www.bbc.com/future/article/20210210-why-the-entire-coronavirus-would-fit-in-a-can-of-coca-cola

3. https://www.thelancet.com/journals/lancet/article/PIIS0140-6736(21)00869-2/fulltext

4. https://www.acpjournals.org/doi/full/10.7326/M20-5008?journalCode=aim&#r61-M205008

5. Meyerowitz EA, Richterman A, Gandhi RT, Sax PE. Transmission of SARS-CoV-2: a review of viral, host, and environmental factors. Annals of internal medicine. 2020 Sep 17

6. https://www.nature.com/articles/d41586-020-03141-3

7. https://www.thelancet.com/journals/lanmic/article/PIIS2666-5247(20)30172-5/fulltext

8. https://journals.plos.org/plosone/article?id=10.1371/journal.pone.0242128

9. https://www.ncbi.nlm.nih.gov/pmc/articles/PMC7338915/
10. https://www.ncbi.nlm.nih.gov/pmc/articles/PMC7338915/
11. https://www.cdc.gov/mmwr/volumes/69/wr/mm6919e6.htm
12. https://jamanetwork.com/journals/jamanetworkopen/fullarticle/2774102
13. https://www.gov.uk/guidance/the-r-number-in-the-uk
14. https://sph.umich.edu/pursuit/2020posts/how-scientists-quantify-outbreaks.html
15. https://science.sciencemag.org/content/369/6505/846/tab-figures-data

---

CHAPTER 4: WHAT IS THE RISK FROM NEW VARIANTS?

1. https://www.gov.uk/government/publications/covid-19-variants-genomically-confirmed-case-numbers/variants-distribution-of-cases-data
2. https://www.theguardian.com/world/2020/dec/20/fast-spreading-covid-variant-in-england-uk
3. https://www.who.int/en/activities/tracking-SARS-CoV-2-variants/
4. https://www.reuters.com/investigates/special-report/health-coronavirus-uk-variant/
5. https://www.gov.uk/government/publications/covid-19-variants-genomically-confirmed-case-numbers/variants-distribution-of-cases-data
6. https://science.sciencemag.org/content/early/2021/03/03/science.abg3055
7. https://www.nature.com/articles/s41586-021-03426-1
8. https://assets.publishing.service.gov.uk/government/uploads/system/uploads/attachment_data/file/972247/Variants_of_Concern_VOC_Technical_Briefing_7_England.pdf
9. https://files.ssi.dk/covid19/virusvarianter/status/status-virusvarianter-04032021-11kk
10. https://assets.publishing.service.gov.uk/government/uploads/system/uploads/attachment_data/file/961299/Variants_of_ConcerN_VOC_Technical_Briefing_6_England-1.pdf
11. https://assets.publishing.service.gov.uk/government/uploads/system/uploads/attachment_data/file/990339/Variants_of_Concern_VOC_Technical_Briefing_13_England.pdf
12. https://www.gisaid.org/index.php?id=208

CHAPTER 5: HOW GOOD ARE DIAGNOSTIC TESTS?

1. https://www.genome.gov/about-genomics/fact-sheets/Polymerase-Chain-Reaction-Fact-Sheet
2. https://assets.publishing.service.gov.uk/government/uploads/system/uploads/attachment_data/file/926410/Understanding_Cycle_Threshold__Ct__iN_SARS-CoV-2_RT-PCR_.pdf
3. https://www.thelancet.com/journals/lanmic/article/PIIS2666-5247(20)30172-5/fulltext
4. https://www.medrxiv.org/content/10.1101/2020.07.10.20150524v1
5. https://www.medrxiv.org/content/10.1101/2020.10.25.20219048v2
6. https://www.medrxiv.org/content/10.1101/2020.10.25.20219048v2
7. https://www.gov.uk/government/publications/sars-cov-2-rna-testing-assurance-of-positive-results-during-periods-of-low-prevalence/assurance-of-sars-cov-2-rna-positive-results-during-periods-of-low-prevalence
8. https://www.ncbi.nlm.nih.gov/pmc/articles/PMC4986465/
9. https://www.thelancet.com/journals/lanpub/article/PIIS2468-2667(20)30282-6/fulltext
10. https://www.medrxiv.org/content/10.1101/2020.10.25.20219048v2
11. https://www.cochranelibrary.com/cdsr/doi/10.1002/14651858.CD013705.pub2/epdf/abstract
12. https://www.gov.uk/government/publications/lateral-flow-device-specificity-in-phase-4-post-marketing-surveillance
13. https://www.huffingtonpost.co.uk/entry/false-positives-coronavirus_uk_5f686da4c5b6de79b677e909

CHAPTER 6: HOW MANY CASES HAVE BEEN FOUND?

1. https://ourworldindata.org/explorers/coronavirus-data-explorer
2. https://www.bbc.co.uk/news/world-africa-54603689
3. https://www.gov.uk/government/publications/weekly-statistics-for-nhs-test-and-trace-england-29-april-to-5-may-2021
4. https://coronavirus.data.gov.uk/details/testing?areaType=nation&areaName=England
5. https://ourworldindata.org/coronavirus-testing
6. https://www.gov.uk/government/publications/sars-cov-2-rna-testing-assurance-of-positive-results-during-periods-of-low-prevalence/

assurance-of-sars-cov-2-rna-positive-results-during-periods-of-low-prevalence

7. https://coronavirus.data.gov.uk/details/about-data#england

CHAPTER 7: HOW MANY PEOPLE HAVE BEEN INFECTED WITH SARS-COV-2?

1. https://blog.ons.gov.uk/2020/05/14/new-survey-results-provide-first-snapshot-of-the-current-number-of-covid-19-infections-in-england/

2. https://www.ons.gov.uk/peoplepopulationandcommunity/health andsocialcare/conditionsanddiseases/datasets/covid19infection surveytechnicaldata

3. https://www.ons.gov.uk/aboutus/transparencyandgovernance/ freedomofinformationfoi/dispatchofvouchersforthecovid19infectionsurvey

4. https://www.ons.gov.uk/peoplepopulationandcommunity/healthand socialcare/conditionsanddiseases/methodologies/covid19infection surveypilotmethodsandfurtherinformation

5. https://www.imperial.ac.uk/medicine/research-and-impact/groups/react-study/the-react-1-programme/

6. https://covid.joinzoe.com/

7. https://www.thelancet.com/journals/lanpub/article/PIIS2468-2667(20)30282-6/fulltext

8. https://www.ons.gov.uk/peoplepopulationandcommunity/health andsocialcare/conditionsanddiseases/articles/coronaviruscovid19 infectionsinthecommunityinengland/characteristicsofpeople testingpositiveforcovid19inengland22february2021#likelihood-of-testing-positive-for-covid-19-by-occupation

9. https://coronavirus.data.gov.uk/details/cases?areaType=nation&areaName=England

10. https://www.ons.gov.uk/peoplepopulationandcommunity/ healthandsocialcare/conditionsanddiseases/articles/coronaviruscovid19inf ectionsurveyantibodydatafortheuk/28april2021

11. https://blog.ons.gov.uk/2021/04/28/antibodies-and-immunity-how-do-they-relate-to-one-another/

12. https://www.bmj.com/content/370/bmj.m3563

13. https://www.mrc-bsu.cam.ac.uk/now-casting/nowcasting-and-forecasting-27th-may-2021/

CHAPTER 8: HOW ILL DO PEOPLE GET WITH COVID-19?

1. https://www.ons.gov.uk/peoplepopulationandcommunity/health andsocialcare/conditionsanddiseases/articles/coronaviruscovid19 infectioninthecommunityinengland/characteristicsofpeopletesting positiveforcovid19incountriesoftheuk5may2021

2. https://evidence.nihr.ac.uk/themedreview/living-with-covid19-second-review/

3. https://www.bbc.co.uk/sounds/play/m000mzms

4. https://www.medrxiv.org/content/10.1101/2021.03.03.21252086v1

5. https://www.ons.gov.uk/peoplepopulationandcommunity/ healthandsocialcare/conditionsanddiseases/bulletins/ prevalenceofongoingsymptomsfollowingcoronaviruscovid19 infectionintheuk/1april2021

6. https://www.nice.org.uk/guidance/ng188/evidence

CHAPTER 9: WHAT HAPPENED IN HOSPITALS?

1. https://www.bbc.co.uk/news/health-51214864

2. https://www.sciencemag.org/news/2020/04/how-does-coronavirus-kill-clinicians-trace-ferocious-rampage-through-body-brain-toes

3. https://www.theguardian.com/world/2020/mar/13/italian-doctor-an-experience-i-would-compare-to-a-world-war

4. https://www.ecdc.europa.eu/en/publications-data/download-data-hospital-and-icu-admission-rates-and-current-occupancy-covid-19

5. https://ourworldindata.org/grapher/weekly-hospital-admissions-covid-per-million?country=GBR~USA~ESP~ITA

6. https://digital.nhs.uk/data-and-information/supplementary-information/2021/hospital-admissions-from-2018-19-to-2020-21

7. https://assets.publishing.service.gov.uk/government/uploads/system/ uploads/attachment_data/file/982289/Weekly_Flu_anD_COVID-19_report_w17.pdf

8. https://www.london.gov.uk/press-releases/mayoral/hospitals-at-risk-of-being-overwhelmed-in-capital

9. https://www.bmj.com/content/372/bmj.n471

10. https://www.england.nhs.uk/statistics/statistical-work-areas/rtt-waiting-times/rtt-data-2021-22/#Apr21

11. https://www.health.org.uk/publications/long-reads/nhs-performance-and-waiting-times

12. https://www.boa.ac.uk/resources/bods-boa-survey-of-impact-of-covid-19-on-uk-orthopaedic-practice-and-implications-on-restoration-of-elective-services-part-2.html

13. https://www.theguardian.com/world/2020/may/04/london-nhs-nightingale-hospital-placed-on-standby

14. https://www.hsj.co.uk/finance-and-efficiency/revealed-nightingale-hospitals-to-cost-half-a-billion-pounds-in-total/7029345.article

15. https://assets.publishing.service.gov.uk/government/uploads/system/uploads/attachment_data/file/943174/S0919_Changes_in_hospital_mortality_in_the_first_wave_oF_COVID-19.pdf

16. https://www.england.nhs.uk/statistics/statistical-work-areas/covid-19-hospital-activity/

17. https://www.icnarc.org/Our-Audit/Audits/Cmp/Reports

18. https://commonslibrary.parliament.uk/research-briefings/sn03336/

19. Michael Rosen p 22 of Many Different Kinds of Love

20. https://www.bmj.com/content/372/bmj.n693

21. https://jamanetwork.com/journals/jama/fullarticle/2774380

22. https://jamanetwork.com/journals/jama/fullarticle/2773128

23. https://fullfact.org/health/coronavirus-transmission-hospitals/

24. https://www.theguardian.com/society/2021/mar/26/40600-people-likely-caught-covid-while-hospital-inpatients-in-england

CHAPTER 10: HOW GOOD ARE THE TREATMENTS FOR COVID-19?

1. https://www.gov.uk/government/news/ventilator-challenge-hailed-a-success-as-uk-production-finishes

2. https://www.icnarc.org/our-audit/audits/cmp/reports

3. https://coronavirusexplained.ukri.org/en/article/vdt0008/

4. https://www.thelancet.com/journals/eclinm/article/PIIS2589-5370(20)30323-0/fulltext

5. https://www.thelancet.com/journals/lanres/article/PIIS2213-2600(20)30581-6/fulltext

6. https://royalpapworth.nhs.uk/our-hospital/latest-news/ECMO-COVID19-coronavirus

7. https://www.timesofisrael.com/madagascar-president-claims-country-develops-herbal-tea-remedy-for-coronavirus/

8. https://www.chicagotribune.com/coronavirus/ct-nw-trump-white-house-sunlight-heat-fight-virus-20200424-7dnhtyxltvdazkp24mybuefmou-story.html

9. https://www.thelancet.com/journals/lancet/article/PIIS0140-6736(20)31958-9/fulltext

10. https://www.bbc.co.uk/news/world-us-canada-53911565

11. https://www.recoverytrial.net/

12. https://www.ncbi.nlm.nih.gov/pmc/articles/PMC7383595/

13. https://www.england.nhs.uk/2021/03/covid-treatment-developed-in-the-nhs-saves-a-million-lives/

14. https://www.thelancet.com/journals/lancet/article/PIIS0140-6736(21)00676-0/fulltext

15. https://www.nejm.org/doi/full/10.1056/NEJMoa2022926

16. https://www.thelancet.com/journals/lancet/article/PIIS0140-6736(21)00897-7/fulltext

17. https://www.health.harvard.edu/diseases-and-conditions/treatments-for-covid-19

18. https://www.fda.gov/consumers/consumer-updates/why-you-should-not-use-ivermectin-treat-or-prevent-covid-19

CHAPTER 11: HOW MANY PEOPLE HAVE DIED FROM COVID-19?

1. https://www.who.int/classifications/icd/Guidelines_Cause_of_DeatH_COVID-19.pdf?ua=1

2. https://www.rivm.nl/coronavirus-covid-19/grafieken

3. https://epistat.wiv-isp.be/Covid/

4. https://www.cdc.gov/coronavirus/2019-ncov/cases-updates/about-us-cases-deaths.html

5. In Wales, Public Health Wales https://public.tableau.com/profile/public.health.wales.health.protection#!/vizhome/RapIDCOVID-19virology-Public/Headlinesummary has three criteria for a COVID-19 death:

    • **Lab-confirmation:** the person must have a positive test result for SARS-CoV-2.

- **Clinical suspicion:** clinicians must suspect that COVID-19 was a causative factor in the death.
- **Location:** the death must occur in a Welsh hospital or care home.

For Scotland (https://www.gov.scot/publications/coronavirus-covid-19-data-definitions-and-sources) and Northern Ireland (https://www.publichealth.hscni.net/publications/covid-19-surveillance-reports), the measure is identical: deaths within 28 days of a positive test for SARS-CoV-2.

6. https://publichealthmatters.blog.gov.uk/2021/02/08/counting-deaths-during-the-pandemic/

7. https://www.gov.uk/government/publications/phe-data-series-on-deaths-in-people-with-covid-19-technical-summary

8. https://www.cebm.net/covid-19/why-no-one-can-ever-recover-from-covid-19-in-england-a-statistical-anomaly/

9. https://www.theguardian.com/world/2020/jul/17/matt-hancock-calls-urgent-inquiry-phe-covid-19-death-figures

10. https://assets.publishing.service.gov.uk/government/uploads/system/uploads/attachment_data/file/916035/RA_Technical_Summary_-_PHE_Data_Series_COVID_19_Deaths_20200812.pdf

11. https://assets.publishing.service.gov.uk/government/uploads/system/uploads/attachment_data/file/877302/guidance-for-doctors-completing-medical-certificates-of-cause-of-death-covid-19.pdf

12. https://www.ons.gov.uk/peoplepopulationandcommunity/birthsdeathsandmarriages/deaths/bulletins/deathsinvolvingcovid19englandandwales/deathsoccurringinjune2020

13. https://www.ons.gov.uk/peoplepopulationandcommunity/birthsdeathsandmarriages/deaths/articles/analysisofdeathregistrationsnotinvolvingcoronaviruscovid19englandandwales28december2019to1may2020/technicalannex#possible-explanations-for-non-covid-19-excess-deaths

14. https://health.org.uk/news-and-comment/news/1.5-million-potential-years-of-life-lost-to-covid-19

15. https://www.nature.com/articles/s41598-021-83040-3

16. https://www.ons.gov.uk/peoplepopulationandcommunity/birthsdeathsandmarriages/deaths/datasets/weeklyprovisionalfiguresondeathsregisteredinenglandandwales

17. https://www.ons.gov.uk/peoplepopulationandcommunity/birthsdeathsandmarriages/deaths/bulletins/deathsregisteredweeklyinenglandandwalesprovisional/weekending14may2021

18. https://www.ons.gov.uk/peoplepopulationandcommunity/birthsdeath
    sandmarriages/deaths/bulletins/deathsinvolvingcovid19englandandwales/
    deathsoccurringinjune2020
19. https://www.ons.gov.uk/peoplepopulationandcommunity/birthsdeathsand
    marriages/deaths/articles/deathsathomeincreasedbyathirdin
    2020whiledeathsinhospitalsfellexceptforcovid19/2021-05-07

CHAPTER 12: HOW LETHAL IS SARS-COV-2?

1. https://www.nhs.uk/conditions/vaccinations/child-flu-vaccine/
2. https://www.imperial.ac.uk/mrc-global-infectious-disease-analysis/
    covid-19/report-34-ifr/
3. https://www.medrxiv.org/content/10.1101/2021.01.15.21249756v2

CHAPTER 13: WHO HAS BEEN MOST AT RISK FROM COVID-19?

1. https://www.ons.gov.uk/peoplepopulationandcommunity/birthsdeathsand
    marriages/deaths/articles/updatingethniccontrastsindeathsinvolvingthe
    coronaviruscovid19englandandwales/deathsoccurring2marchto28july2020
2. https://www.ons.gov.uk/peoplepopulationandcommunity/birthsdeathsand
    marriages/deaths/articles/updatingethniccontrastsindeathsinvolvingthe
    coronaviruscovid19englandandwales/24january2020to31march2021
3. https://www.nature.com/articles/s41467-021-21237-w
4. https://www.ethnicity-facts-figures.service.gov.uk/housing/housing-
    conditions/overcrowded-households/latest
5. https://www.thelancet.com/journals/lancet/article/PIIS0140-6736(21)
    00634-6/fulltext
6. https://www.ons.gov.uk/peoplepopulationandcommunity/
    healthandsocialcare/causesofdeath/bulletins/
    coronaviruscovid19relateddeathsbyoccupationenglandandwales/
    deathsregisteredbetween9marchand28december2020
7. https://committees.parliament.uk/work/1003/covid19-supporting-the-
    vulnerable-during-lockdown
8. https://www.nature.com/articles/s41586-020-2521-4
9. https://alama.org.uk/covid-19-medical-risk-assessment/
10. https://qcovid.org/Calculation

11. https://www.bmj.com/content/372/bmj.n467
12. https://digital.nhs.uk/coronavirus/risk-assessment/population
13. https://www.thelancet.com/journals/lanepe/article/PIIS2666-7762(21) 00086-7/fulltext

CHAPTER 14: HOW DO WE COMPARE COUNTRIES?

1. https://odihpn.org/resources/interpreting-and-using-mortality-data-in-humanitarian-emergencies/
2. https://assets.publishing.service.gov.uk/government/uploads/system/uploads/attachment_data/file/957265/s0980-direct-indirect-impacts-covid-19-excess-deaths-morbidity-sage-december-update-final.pdf
3. https://fingertips.phe.org.uk/static-reports/mortality-surveillance/excess-mortality-in-england-latest.html
4. https://www.euromomo.eu/how-it-works/methods/
5. https://www.cdc.gov/nchs/nvss/vsrr/covid19/excess_deaths.htm
6. https://www.ncbi.nlm.nih.gov/pmc/articles/PMC7852240/
7. https://ec.europa.eu/eurostat/web/population-demography-migration-projections/data/main-tables
8. https://www.nrscotland.gov.uk/files/statistics/age-standardised-death-rates-esp/age-standard-death-rates-background.pdf
9. https://www.opendata.nhs.scot/dataset/standard-populations
10. https://www.ons.gov.uk/peoplepopulationandcommunity/births deathsandmarriages/deaths/articles/comparisonsofallcausemortality betweeneuropeancountriesandregions/2020
11. https://www.theguardian.com/commentisfree/2020/apr/30/coronavirus-deaths-how-does-britain-compare-with-other-countries

CHAPTER 15: HOW DOES THE IMPACT OF COVID-19 COMPARE WITH OTHER HISTORICAL HARMS?

1. https://journals.plos.org/plosone/article?id=10.1371/journal.pone.0242128
2. https://bmcinfectdis.biomedcentral.com/articles/10.1186/1471-2334-14-480
3. https://www.economist.com/graphic-detail/2020/09/12/the-southern-hemisphere-skipped-flu-season-in-2020

4. https://www.who.int/docs/default-source/coronaviruse/situation-reports/
    20200306-sitrep-46-covid-19.pdf?sfvrsn=96b04adf_4

5. https://assets.publishing.service.gov.uk/government/uploads/system/
    uploads/attachment_data/file/895233/Surveillance_Influenza_and_other_
    respiratory_viruses_in_the_UK_2019_to_2020_FINAL.pdf

6. https://www.nomisweb.co.uk/

7. https://www.ons.gov.uk/peoplepopulationandcommunity/births
    deathsandmarriages/deaths/datasets/weeklyprovisionalfigureson
    deathsregisteredinenglandandwales

8. https://www.ons.gov.uk/peoplepopulationandcommunity/birthsdeaths
    andmarriages/deaths/bulletins/monthlymortalityanalysisenglandandwales/
    april2021

9. https://www.nomisweb.co.uk/query/construct/summary.asp?mode=constr
    uct&version=0&dataset=161

10. https://www.ons.gov.uk/peoplepopulationandcommunity/birthsdeaths
    andmarriages/deaths/adhocs/12735annualdeathsandmortalityrates1938to
    2020provisional

11. https://ourworldindata.org/life-expectancy

CHAPTER 16: WHAT IS THE EFFECT OF MEASURES AGAINST
THE SPREAD OF SARS-COV-2?

1. https://www.thelancet.com/journals/lancet/article/PIIS0140-6736(21)
    00978-8/fulltext

2. https://www.acpjournals.org/doi/10.7326/M20-6817

3. https://www.bmj.com/content/371/bmj.m4586

4. https://www.bsg.ox.ac.uk/research/research-projects/covid-19-government-
    response-tracker

5. https://www.nature.com/articles/s41586-020-2405-7

6. https://www.nature.com/articles/s41586-020-3025-y

7. https://bmcmedicine.biomedcentral.com/articles/10.1186/s12916-020-
    01872-8

8. https://science.sciencemag.org/content/371/6531/eabd9338

9. https://www.ons.gov.uk/peoplepopulationandcommunity/
    healthandsocialcare/conditionsanddiseases/bulletins/coronaviruscovid1
    9infectionsurveypilot/9april2021#number-of-new-covid-19-infections-in-
    england-wales-northern-ireland-and-scotland

10. https://www.medrxiv.org/content/10.1101/2021.01.11.21249564v1

11. https://www.gov.uk/government/publications/npis-table-17-september-2020
12. https://ourworldindata.org/grapher/international-travel-covid
13. https://www.ons.gov.uk/peoplepopulationandcommunity/
    leisureandtourism/bulletins/overseastravelandtourism/apriltojune2020
14. https://www.gov.uk/government/publications/sage-minutes-coronavirus-
    covid-19-response-3-february-2020/sage-3-minutes-coronavirus-covid-19-
    response-3-february-2020
15. https://www.thelancet.com/journals/lanpub/article/PIIS2468-2667(20)
    30263-2/fulltext
16. https://www.gov.uk/government/publications/cog-uk-impact-of-travel-
    restrictions-on-importations-to-england-from-may-to-september-2020-16-
    march-2021
17. https://www.who.int/news-room/q-a-detail/contact-tracing
18. https://www.bbc.co.uk/news/world-asia-53620633
19. https://www.gov.uk/government/publications/weekly-statistics-for-nhs-
    test-and-trace-england-29-april-to-5-may-2021
20. https://www.ons.gov.uk/peoplepopulationandcommunity/healthand
    socialcare/healthandwellbeing/bulletins/coronavirusandselfisolation
    aftertestingpositiveinengland/12aprilto16april2021
21. https://assets.publishing.service.gov.uk/government/uploads/system/
    uploads/attachment_data/file/986380/Variants_of_Concern_VOC_
    Technical_Briefing_11_England.pdf
22. https://assets.publishing.service.gov.uk/government/uploads/system/
    uploads/attachment_data/file/960110/RUM_model_technical_annex_
    final__100221.pdf
23. https://www.nhs.uk/apps-library/nhs-covid-19/
24. https://www.nature.com/articles/s41586-021-03606-z

CHAPTER 17: WHAT HAVE BEEN THE COLLATERAL EFFECTS OF THE MEASURES AGAINST COVID-19?

1. https://www.sciencedirect.com/science/article/pii/S0140673620313568
2. https://www.health.org.uk/news-and-comment/charts-and-infographics/
   exploring-the-fall-in-a-e-visits-during-the-pandemic
3. https://drfoster.com/2020/10/14/quantifying-nhs-activity-reduction-
   during-the-peak-of-the-covid-19-crisis/
4. https://news.cancerresearchuk.org/2021/03/11/2000-fewer-people-in-
   england-began-cancer-treatment-in-january/

5. https://app.powerbi.com/view?r=eyJrIjoiYmUwNmFhMjYtNGZhYSoo
    NDk2LWFlMTAtOTgoOGNhNmFiNGMoIiwidCI6ImVlNGUxNDk5
    LTRhMzUtNGIyZS1hZDQ3LTVmM2NmOWRlODY2NiIsImMiOjh9

6. https://www.cdc.gov/mmwr/volumes/69/wr/mm6937a6.htm

7. https://www.gov.uk/government/statistics/national-flu-and-covid-19-
    surveillance-reports

8. https://www.gov.uk/government/statistical-data-sets/ras45-quarterly-
    statistics#monthly-trends

9. https://injuryprevention.bmj.com/content/27/1/98

10. https://www.nationalgeographic.com/animals/article/coronavirus-
    pandemic-fake-animal-viral-social-media-posts

11. https://analytics.phe.gov.uk/apps/covid-19-indirect-effects/

12. https://www.bbc.com/future/article/20200506-why-lockdown-is-helping-
    bees

13. https://www.bbc.com/future/article/20210312-covid-19-paused-climate-
    emissions-but-theyre-rising-again

14. https://www.bmj.com/content/372/bmj.n521

CHAPTER 18: HOW HAS BEHAVIOUR CHANGED DURING THE PANDEMIC?

1. https://www.ons.gov.uk/peoplepopulationandcommunity/
    healthandsocialcare/healthandwellbeing/bulletins/coronavirusandthesocia
    limpactsongreatbritain/14may2021

2. https://www.ons.gov.uk/peoplepopulationandcommunity/crimeandjustice/
    bulletins/crimeinenglandandwales/yearendingseptember2020

3. https://news.npcc.police.uk/releases/update-on-national-crime-trends-
    and-fixed-penalty-notices-issued-under-covid-regulations

4. https://www.gov.uk/government/statistics/police-powers-and-procedures-
    england-and-wales-year-ending-31-march-2020

5. https://www.gov.uk/government/speeches/pm-statement-on-coronavirus-
    16-march-2020

6. https://blog.zoom.us/90-day-security-plan-progress-report-april-22/

7. https://www.microsoft.com/en-us/microsoft-365/blog/2020/10/28/
    microsoft-teams-reaches-115-million-dau-plus-a-new-daily-collaboration-
    minutes-metric-for-microsoft-365/

8. https://support.google.com/covid19-mobility/answer/9824897?hl=en&ref_
    topic=9822927

9. https://ourworldindata.org/covid-mobility-trends
10. https://analytics.phe.gov.uk/apps/covid-19-indirect-effects/
11. https://www.sheffield.ac.uk/news/new-study-reveals-how-first-lockdown-impacted-alcohol-consumption
12. http://www.alcoholinengland.info/index
13. https://www.gov.uk/government/statistics/alcohol-bulletin/alcohol-bulletin-commentary-november-2020-to-january-2021
14. https://analytics.phe.gov.uk/apps/covid-19-indirect-effects/#
15. https://www.sportengland.org/know-your-audience/data/active-lives
16. https://www.ons.gov.uk/economy/environmentalaccounts/articles/howhaslockdownchangedourrelationshipwithnature/2021-04-26
17. https://www.emcdda.europa.eu/publications/ad-hoc/covid-19-and-drugs-drug-supply-via-darknet-markets_en
18. https://www.ons.gov.uk/peoplepopulationandcommunity/crimeandjustice/bulletins/crimeinenglandandwales/yearendingseptember2020
19. https://www.met.police.uk/sd/stats-and-data/met/stop-and-search-dashboard/
20. https://www.ons.gov.uk/peoplepopulationandcommunity/crimeandjustice/articles/domesticabuseduringthecoronaviruscovid19pandemicenglandandwales/november2020
21. https://www.refuge.org.uk/a-year-of-lockdown/
22. https://www.gov.uk/government/news/home-secretary-announces-support-for-domestic-abuse-victims
23. https://www.pornhub.com/insights/coronavirus-update-april-14

CHAPTER 19: WHAT HAS HAPPENED TO MENTAL HEALTH AND WELL-BEING?

1. https://www.ons.gov.uk/peoplepopulationandcommunity/healthandsocialcare/healthandlifeexpectancies/methodologies/opinionsandlifestylesurveyqmi
2. https://www.ons.gov.uk/peoplepopulationandcommunity/healthandsocialcare/healthandwellbeing/bulletins/coronavirusandthesocialimpactsongreatbritain/12march2021
3. https://www.ons.gov.uk/peoplepopulationandcommunity/wellbeing/articles/measuringnationalwellbeing/internationalcomparisons2019
4. https://www.ons.gov.uk/peoplepopulationandcommunity/wellbeing/articles/coronavirusanddepressioninadultsgreatbritain/june2020

5. https://www.ons.gov.uk/peoplepopulationandcommunity/wellbeing/articles/mappinglonelinessduringthecoronaviruspandemic/2021-04-07

6. https://www.itv.com/news/2020-05-06/charity-warns-of-mental-illness-timebomb-as-calls-increase-by-200

7. https://fullfact.org/online/suicide-200-percent/

8. https://www.ons.gov.uk/peoplepopulationandcommunity/birthsdeathsandmarriages/deaths/bulletins/quarterlysuicidedeathregistrationsinengland/2001to2019registrationsandquarter1jantomartoquarter3julytosept2020provisionaldata

9. https://www.thelancet.com/journals/lanepe/article/PIIS2666-7762(21)00087-9/fulltext

10. https://www.thelancet.com/journals/lanpsy/article/PIIS2215-0366(21)00091-2/fulltext

---

CHAPTER 20: WHAT HAVE BEEN PEOPLE'S ATTITUDES AND BELIEFS ABOUT THE PANDEMIC?

1. https://www.tandfonline.com/doi/full/10.1080/13669877.2021.1890637
   They questioned over 1,000 (different) people at five different times over 2020. DS was a collaborator on this study.

2. https://www.ons.gov.uk/peoplepopulationandcommunity/healthandsocialcare/healthandwellbeing/bulletins/coronavirusandthesocialimpactsongreatbritain/30april2021

3. https://www.ipsos.com/ipsos-mori/en-uk/most-britons-continue-say-they-are-following-coronavirus-rules-almost-half-believe-lockdown

4. https://www.ipsos.com/ipsos-mori/en-uk/ukri-research-how-has-covid-19-affected-trust-scientists 11,646 online UK adults aged 16 and over interviewed from 10 April to 17 August 2020.

5. https://www.ipsos.com/sites/default/files/ct/news/documents/2021-03/one_year_covid19_institutions_.pdf

6. https://gh.bmj.com/content/5/5/e002604

7. https://www.nature.com/articles/s41562-021-01056-1

8. https://www.who.int/emergencies/diseases/novel-coronavirus-2019/advice-for-public/myth-busters

9. https://royalsocietypublishing.org/doi/10.1098/rsos.201199

CHAPTER 21: WHAT HAS BEEN THE EFFECT ON THE ECONOMY?

1. https://www.gov.uk/government/speeches/pm-statement-on-coronavirus-16-march-2020
2. https://www.gov.uk/guidance/claim-for-wages-through-the-coronavirus-job-retention-scheme
3. https://www.ons.gov.uk/employmentandlabourmarket/peopleinwork/employmentandemployeetypes/bulletins/employmentintheuk/february2021
4. https://www.ons.gov.uk/economy/grossdomesticproductgdp/bulletins/quarterlynationalaccounts/julytoseptember2020
5. https://osr.statisticsauthority.gov.uk/correspondence/ed-humpherson-to-simon-briscoe-concerns-regarding-ons-gdp-statistics-during-the-pandemic/
6. https://www.ons.gov.uk/economy/grossdomesticproductgdp/articles/internationalcomparisonsofgdpduringthecoronaviruscovid19pandemic/2021-02-01
7. https://www.ons.gov.uk/economy/governmentpublicsectorandtaxes/publicsectorfinance/bulletins/publicsectorfinances/march2021
8. https://www.ons.gov.uk/businessindustryandtrade/retailindustry/bulletins/retailsales/january2021
9. https://blog.ons.gov.uk/2020/06/29/shopping-may-never-be-the-same-again/
10. https://www.nytimes.com/2021/04/29/technology/amazons-profits-triple.html
11. https://www.ons.gov.uk/businessindustryandtrade/retailindustry/timeseries/ms72/drsi
12. https://s22.q4cdn.com/959853165/files/doc_financials/2020/q4/FINAL-Q420-Shareholder-Letter.pdf
13. https://www.cnbc.com/2021/02/11/disney-dis-q1-2021-earnings.html
14. https://www.nintendo.co.jp/ir/en/finance/hard_soft/number.html

CHAPTER 22: HOW EFFECTIVE ARE THE VACCINES?

1. https://www.raps.org/news-and-articles/news-articles/2020/3/covid-19-vaccine-tracker

2. https://www.bbc.co.uk/news/health-54902908
3. https://www.nice.org.uk/glossary?letter=r
4. https://www.gsk.com/en-gb/research-and-development/trials-in-people/clinical-trial-phases/
5. https://www.who.int/influenza_vaccines_plan/resources/Session4_VEfficacy_VEffectiveness.PDF
6. https://www.nejm.org/doi/full/10.1056/nejmoa2034577
7. https://xkcd.com/2400/
8. https://www.nejm.org/doi/full/10.1056/NEJMoa2034577
9. https://www.astrazeneca.com/media-centre/press-releases/2021/azd1222-us-phase-iii-primary-analysis-confirms-safety-and-efficacy.html
10. https://www.nejm.org/doi/full/10.1056/nejmoa2035389
11. https://www.thelancet.com/journals/lancet/article/PIIS0140-6736(21)00234-8/fulltext
12. https://ir.novavax.com/news-releases/news-release-details/novavax-confirms-high-levels-efficacy-against-original-and-0
13. https://www.cdc.gov/mmwr/volumes/70/wr/mm7009e4.htm?s_cid=mm7009e4_w
14. https://apps.who.int/iris/bitstream/handle/10665/341454/WHO-2019-nCoV-vaccines-SAGE-recommendation-Sinovac-CoronaVac-2021.1-eng.pdf
15. https://www.bmj.com/content/372/bmj.n597
16. https://reason.com/2021/02/23/vaccines-are-100-effective-at-preventing-covid-19-hospitalizations-and-deaths/
17. https://www.bmj.com/content/371/bmj.m4037
18. https://sphweb.bumc.bu.edu/otlt/MPH-Modules/EP/EP713_Cohort Studies/EP713_CohortStudies_print.html
19. https://www.thelancet.com/journals/lancet/article/PIIS0140-6736(21)00677-2/fulltext
20. https://www.nejm.org/doi/full/10.1056/NEJMoa2101765
21. https://www.medrxiv.org/content/10.1101/2021.04.22.21255913v1
22. https://www.gov.uk/government/news/one-dose-of-covid-19-vaccine-can-cut-household-transmission-by-up-to-half
23. https://www.gov.uk/government/publications/investigation-of-novel-sars-cov-2-variant-variant-of-concern-20201201
24. https://www.gov.uk/government/publications/phe-monitoring-of-the-effectiveness-of-covid-19-vaccination
25. https://www.ft.com/content/d71729a3-72e8-490c-bd7e-757027f9b226

CHAPTER 23: HOW SAFE ARE THE VACCINES?

1. https://www.ncbi.nlm.nih.gov/pmc/articles/PMC3136032/
2. https://www.nejm.org/doi/10.1056/NEJMoa021134
3. https://assets.publishing.service.gov.uk/government/uploads/system/uploads/attachment_data/file/963928/UKPAR_COVID_19_Vaccine_AstraZeneca_23.02.2021.pdf
4. https://www.thelancet.com/journals/lancet/article/PIIS0140-6736(20)32661-1/fulltext#supplementaryMaterial
5. https://www.nejm.org/doi/full/10.1056/NEJMoa2034577
6. http://www.histmodbiomed.org/sites/default/files/44823.pdf
7. https://web.archive.org/web/20210507220701/https://www.gov.uk/government/publications/coronavirus-covid-19-vaccine-adverse-reactions/coronavirus-vaccine-summary-of-yellow-card-reporting
8. https://covid.joinzoe.com/post/covid-vaccine-data-lancet
9. https://pubmed.ncbi.nlm.nih.gov/22996960/
10. https://www.nejm.org/doi/full/10.1056/NEJMoa2104840
11. https://britishskydiving.org/how-safe/
12. https://www.nhs.uk/conditions/general-anaesthesia/
13. https://www.ema.europa.eu/en/human-regulatory/post-authorisation/referral-procedures/combined-hormonal-contraceptives
14. https://qualitysafety.bmj.com/content/13/3/176
15. https://www.gov.uk/government/publications/regulatory-approval-of-covid-19-vaccine-astrazeneca/information-for-uk-recipients-on-covid-19-vaccine-astrazeneca#possible-side-effects
    https://www.gov.uk/government/publications/regulatory-approval-of-pfizer-biontech-vaccine-for-covid-19/information-for-uk-recipients-on-pfizerbiontech-covid-19-vaccine#side-effects
16. https://www.fda.gov/news-events/press-announcements/joint-cdc-and-fda-statement-johnson-johnson-covid-19-vaccine

CHAPTER 24: WHO HAS BEEN GETTING THE VACCINES?

1. https://www.reuters.com/article/uk-factcheck-transmission/fact-check-scientists-do-not-yet-know-whether-the-covid-19-vaccine-reduces-transmission-of-the-virus-IDUSKBN29N1UH
2. https://www.gov.uk/government/publications/priority-groups-for-coronavirus-covid-19-vaccination-advice-from-the-jcvi-30-december-2020/

joint-committee-on-vaccination-and-immunisation-advice-on-priority-groups-for-covid-19-vaccination-30-december-2020

3. https://www.sciencedirect.com/science/article/pii/S2666776220300211?via%3Dihub
4. https://www.bmj.com/content/371/bmj.m3731
5. https://www.nature.com/articles/s41586-020-2521-4
6. https://www.gov.uk/government/publications/priority-groups-for-coronavirus-covid-19-vaccination-advice-from-the-jcvi-30-december-2020/joint-committee-on-vaccination-and-immunisation-advice-on-priority-groups-for-covid-19-vaccination-30-december-2020
7. https://www.gov.uk/government/publications/covid-19-response-spring-2021/covid-19-response-spring-2021
8. https://www.opensafely.org/research/2021/covid-vaccine-coverage/
9. https://www.gov.uk/government/publications/priority-groups-for-phase-2-of-the-coronavirus-covid-19-vaccination-programme-advice-from-the-jcvi/jcvi-final-statement-on-phase-2-of-the-covid-19-vaccination-programme-13-april-2021
10. https://www.cdc.gov/coronavirus/2019-ncov/vaccines/recommendations.html
11. https://www.ons.gov.uk/peoplepopulationandcommunity/healthandsocialcare/healthandwellbeing/bulletins/covid19vaccinerefusaluk/februarytomarch2021
12. https://www.ons.gov.uk/peoplepopulationandcommunity/healthandsocialcare/conditionsanddiseases/articles/coronaviruscovid19infectionsurveyantibodydatafortheuk/28april2021

CHAPTER 25: HOW FAR APART SHOULD THE VACCINES BE GIVEN?

1. https://www.washingtonpost.com/world/europe/uk-variant-covid-vaccines/2021/01/26/03533f3a-5ca0-11eb-a849-6f9423a75ffd_story.html
2. https://assets.publishing.service.gov.uk/government/uploads/system/uploads/attachment_data/file/955846/annex-b-comparison-between-1-and-2-dose-prioritisation-for-a-fixed-number-of-doses.pdf
3. https://coronavirus.data.gov.uk/details/vaccinations
4. https://www.science.org.au/learning/immunisation-and-climate-change/science-immunisation/what-is-immunisation

5. https://www.medrxiv.org/content/10.1101/2021.01.30.21250843v5
6. https://www.bmj.com/content/372/bmj.n18
7. https://www.thelancet.com/journals/lancet/article/PIIS0140-6736(21)00432-3/fulltext
8. https://www.nejm.org/doi/full/10.1056/NEJMc2032195
9. https://www.ons.gov.uk/peoplepopulationandcommunity/healthandsocialcare/conditionsanddiseases/articles/coronaviruscovid19infectionsurveyantibodydatafortheuk/13may2021
10. https://assets.publishing.service.gov.uk/government/uploads/system/uploads/attachment_data/file/971017/SP_PH__VE_report_20210317_CC_JLB.pdf
11. https://www.medrxiv.org/content/10.1101/2021.05.15.21257017v1

CHAPTER 26: HOW GOOD ARE THE PROJECTIONS FROM EPIDEMIC MODELS?

1. https://www.bmj.com/about-bmj/resources-readers/publications/epidemiology-uninitiated/1-what-epidemiology
2. https://www.imperial.ac.uk/media/imperial-college/medicine/sph/ide/gida-fellowships/Imperial-College-COVID19-NPI-modelling-16-03-2020.pdf
3. https://arxiv.org/abs/2004.04734
4. https://www.vox.com/future-perfect/2020/5/2/21241261/coronavirus-modeling-us-deaths-ihme-pandemic
5. https://data.chhs.ca.gov/dataset/Covid-19-time-series-metrics-by-county-and-state
6. https://assets.publishing.service.gov.uk/government/uploads/system/uploads/attachment_data/file/958746/S0663_SPI-M-O_Reasonable_worst-case_planning_scenario.pdf
7. https://www.bbc.co.uk/news/health-54831334
8. https://www.gov.uk/government/publications/Covid-19-response-spring-2021
9. https://www.gov.uk/government/publications/spi-m-o-summary-of-modelling-on-roadmap-scenarios-17-february-2021
10. https://journals.plos.org/plosone/article?id=10.1371/journal.pone.0250935
11. https://quoteinvestigator.com/2013/10/20/no-predict/

CHAPTER 27: WHAT IS GOING TO HAPPEN IN THE FUTURE?

1. https://www.scientificamerican.com/article/how-the-covid-19-pandemic-could-end1/
2. https://www.cdc.gov/flu/pandemic-resources/2009-h1n1-pandemic.html
3. https://www.who.int/health-topics/severe-acute-respiratory-syndrome
4. https://assets.publishing.service.gov.uk/government/uploads/system/uploads/attachment_data/file/975909/S1182_SPI-M-O_Summary_of_modelling_of_easing_roadmap_step_2_restrictions.pdf
5. https://www.gov.uk/government/publications/spi-m-o-summary-of-further-modelling-of-easing-restrictions-roadmap-step-3-5-may-2021

CHAPTER 28: POSTSCRIPT

1. https://rss.org.uk/statistics-data-and-covid/

Index

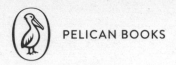

PELICAN BOOKS

Economics:
The User's Guide
Ha-Joon Chang

Human Evolution
Robin Dunbar

Revolutionary Russia:
1891–1991
Orlando Figes

The Domesticated Brain
Bruce Hood

Greek and Roman Political Ideas
Melissa Lane

Classical Literature
Richard Jenkyns

Who Governs Britain?
Anthony King

How to See the World
Nicholas Mirzoeff

The Meaning of Science
Tim Lewens

Social Class in the 21st Century
Mike Savage

The European Union:
A Citizen's Guide
Chris Bickerton

The Caliphate
Hugh Kennedy

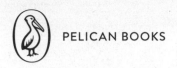

PELICAN BOOKS

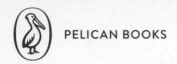

PELICAN BOOKS

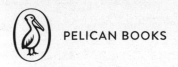

PELICAN BOOKS

Architecture:
From Prehistory to Climate Emergency
Barnabas Calder

Covid by Numbers:
Making Sense of the Pandemic with Data
David Spiegelhalter and Anthony Masters

Around the World in 80 Books
David Damrosch

How Religion Evolved:
And Why It Endures
Robin Dunbar